101 Weight Loss Tips

101 Weight Loss Tips

Dr. Anil Chaturvedi

PRABHAT PRAKASHAN

The diagnosis, treatment and health-related measures/ suggestions given in the book should be consulted with a medical specialist before adopting them.

Published by
PRABHAT PRAKASHAN PVT. LTD.
4/19 Asaf Ali Road,
New Delhi-110 002 (INDIA)
e-mail: prabhatbooks@gmail.com

ISBN 978-93-5186-621-3
101 WEIGHT LOSS TIPS
by Dr. Anil Chaturvedi

Edition
2025

Price
₹ 500.00 (Rupees Five Hundred only)

Printed at
Print Media, New Delhi

Author's Note

Obesity makes it hard even to move around. As you grow in age, lethargy also starts encompassing you along with diseases. The fact is that obesity or increase in weight is caused due to the imbalance in the consumption of energy and its utilization. Another cause of obesity is the intake of fatty food. Obesity is a malady that can inflict any human being.

Agents of Obesity

- Excessive diet, sedentary lifestyle, lack of physical exercise.
- Laziness and not exerting oneself physically.
- Irregular meal timings; diet compromising fat, sweets, oil, ghee, milk, eggs, alcohol, meat; smoking and that too excessively.
- Obesity can be hereditary too. If many people in the family are obese, chances are, the offspring will be obese too.
- As cough and constipation are considered to be the harbingers of disease, similarly is the obesity. It is the origin of many ailments. In fact, the amount of fat keeps increasing in an obese man in comparison to other required by the body. An obese man does not eat to satisfy his hunger; rather, he eats to pacify his taste buds. We can infer that our body starts gathering fat unnecessarily when it gets additional food and rest. Lacks of physical activities contribute to be over-weight.
- Many a times, due to imbalance in behavior and mental tension, people start eating more. As a result, obesity

grasps them. Increased weight introduces an individual to cancer. Obesity can possibly lead to breast and intestinal cancer. Besides this, cancer can make its place in pancreas or kidney also. In both the cases, chances of survival are dim.

Objective of the Book

This book contains a number of utilitarian methods which can help anyone to keep his weight under control and lead a healthy-balanced life.

—Dr. Anil Chaturvedi

Contents

1

Why Perfect Weight is a Necessity?

You are often conscious about your figure, but have you ever worried about your weight? Have you ever tried to ponder whether your weight is in consonance with the various fitness norms? The question is why you should know about the ideal weight of your body? The answer is, on the basis of your ideal weight, you will be able to know if your body is struggling with any of the threatsof health hazards.

Necessity of a Perfect Weight

Perfect weight means having sound body fat in proportion to the body mass, i.e. your weight should be in accordance with your height. If you have a right type of weight, you will appear younger than your actual age and you will easily be able adopt a better lifestyle. On the other hand, being corpulent augments the risk of numerous terrible diseases. In Indian cities, as many as 65% of the youth are either weighty or they are discomfited with their extra weight. Such people are suffering from heart ailments, high blood pressure, type II Diabetes, Osteoarthritis. Some are facing different types of cancers or respiratory ailments. Many are at the threshold of acquiring these diseases.

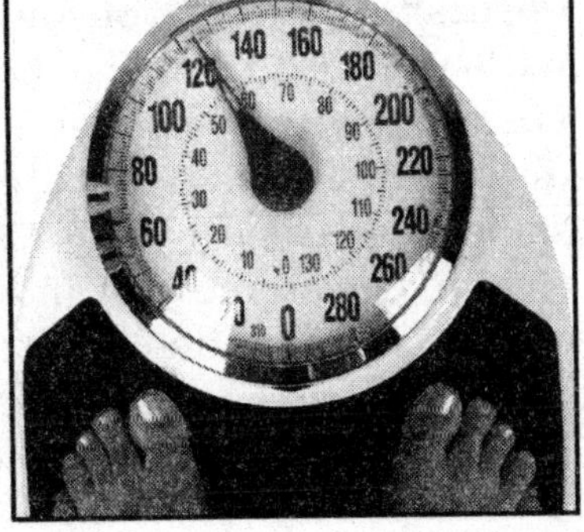

Health specialists consider that BMI (Body Mass Index) is the right scale to measure obesity. Many trainers prefer to measure waist and hip to check the fitness instead of measuring waist only.

Keep a Watch over Body Mass Index (BMI)

If you keep a watch over your BMI, you can conveniently keep your weight under control. If you are overweight then first try to prevent further obesity then it will be easy to tackle the present obesity and reduce it further.

If your BMI range is healthy, you can even increase your weight through balanced diet and exercise.

If your BMI indicates your healthy weight then it becomes all the more important to measure your waist. If your waist measures more than 80 cm then there is a possibility of your lower part of the body gaining fat. Women are more prone to weight gain in the area down the waist. Just stand straight to measure your waist, and measure the area over the hip bones. This needs to be done soon after you release your breath.

Researches reveal that if you have been over weight for a long time then a decrease in your weight by 5 to 15% can result in a spectacular health gain.

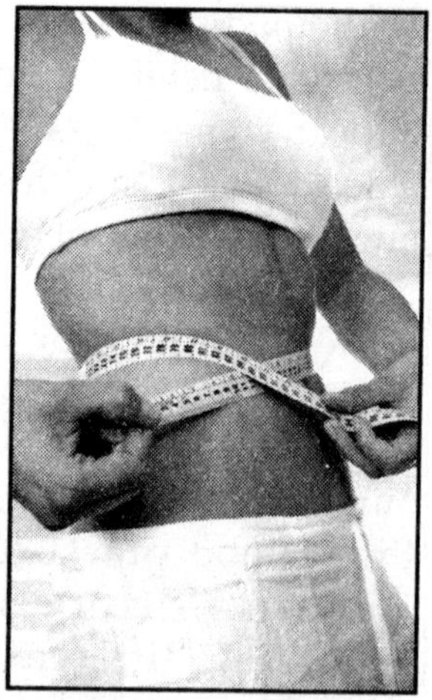

You can check Your BMI This Way

The international Standard to check obesity is BMI i.e. Body Mass Index. To ascertain your BMI, divide your weight (in Kg.) by your height (inches). On the basis of your BMI, you will be able to know whether you posses the ideal weight or if it is more or less than it. According to the standards issued by the Ministry of Health, Government of India, BMI is below 23 is considered normal, more than 25 is rated as overweight while BMI above 25 indicates that a person is suffering somewhere due to obesity.

□

2

Is your Weight Right?

Most of the books dealing with tricks and techniques to lose weight suggest more of protein and fat intake than carbohydrates. The first question that this piece of advice raises in mind is: "How can you lose your weight with diet having more of protein and fat and less of carbohydrate?" You are further advised that one can have eggs in breakfast, dry chapattis in lunch and only soup in dinner.

This advice sounds effective which also suggest that you must exclude carbohydrates from your diet; for example, vegetables, fruits, bread, potato, pasta have been declared 'a

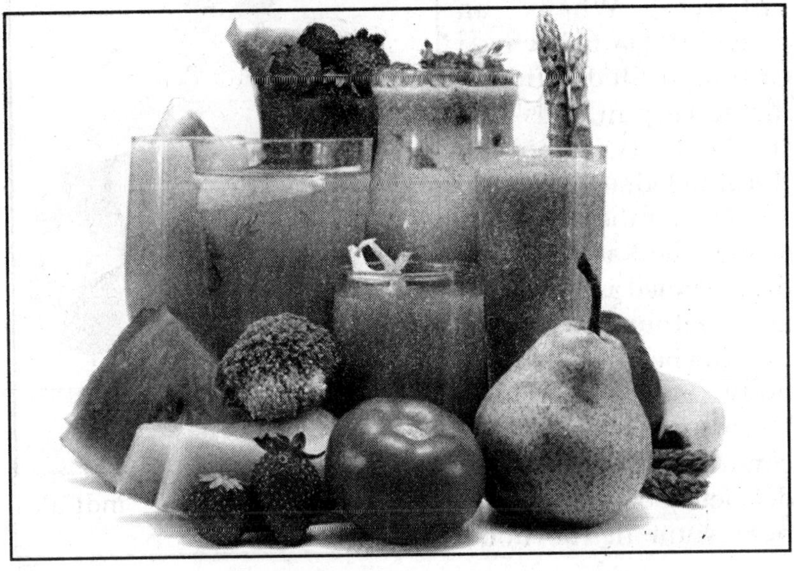

strict no-no'. Does it not sound strange? Of course! This is not right.

It is a fact that less consumption of carbohydrates makes you feel light initially but the weight loss at primary stage is actually the loss of water in the body. It happens due to a metabolic process called ketosis. This procedure is found functional in ailing body (such as those suffering from diabetes or kidney ailments). This is not expected in healthy people. As soon as the body loses water, the consumption of fat begins. This process can be considered apt as far as weight loss is concerned but it has a negative aspect too. The ketosis process leads to destruction of protein in the body also, which can prove disastrous to the body. The body extracts energy by burning protein, which is a vital element of the body and is essential for life (because protein plays a key role in building and maintaining body cells and organs).

This is a well-known fact that when one's urine contains a substance called ketones, it indicates that the cells of your body have started consuming the cells of your muscles. This is the reason that the people who start this diet feel lethargic and listlessness initially. When an individual starts having a carbohydrated efficient diet to keep fit, cells' loss in the body impose a threat to kidney and liver.

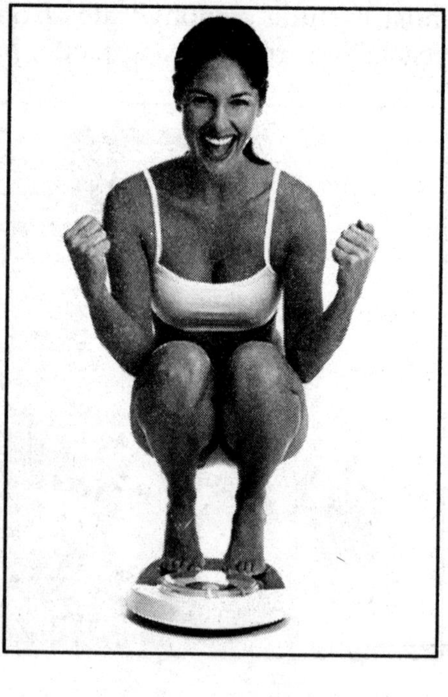

During the process of ketosis, the Katy acid gets disintegrated into ketones and acetones, which in turn can be utilized by the body as a fuel. Unfortunately, this condition often leads to deficiency of sodium and potassium in the body also. Both these minerals play a imperative role in keeping the body healthy. It also brings down the level of thyroid hormone and the body's metabolism starts to conserve energy at a lower rate. It also results into a slower process of weight loss. During the process of ketosis, the amount of blood cholesterol in the body increases, which is quite harmful for health. This process can affect the brain adversely.

Thus, it is visible that this method of weight loss can prove disastrous and continuing with it can result in more harm than good. Besides, as soon as this type of diet is discontinued, the body gains weight at a tremendous rate; as body happens to be in a condition of carbohydrate, water and other nutrients' deficiency. The apostate (the centre in the brain that stimulates hunger) too increases your appetite, and one starts more amount of intake of carbohydrates.

□

3

Deficiency of Carbohydrates is Dangerous!

A research paper was presented in the Annual General Body Meeting of the American College of Preventive Medicine on 21 February, 2004, which revealed: "In the midst of misunderstandings prevailing in the society regarding less intake of carbohydrates in diet to reduce weight is nothing but insanity." This research paper was presented by David L. Kaj, M.D., M.P.H. of Yale Preventive Medicine, Research Centre, Connecticut. This research paper was published in the Medscape Medical News Report, 2004.

This research paper revealed that the diet which does vanishes away the imbalance of energy cannot be considered

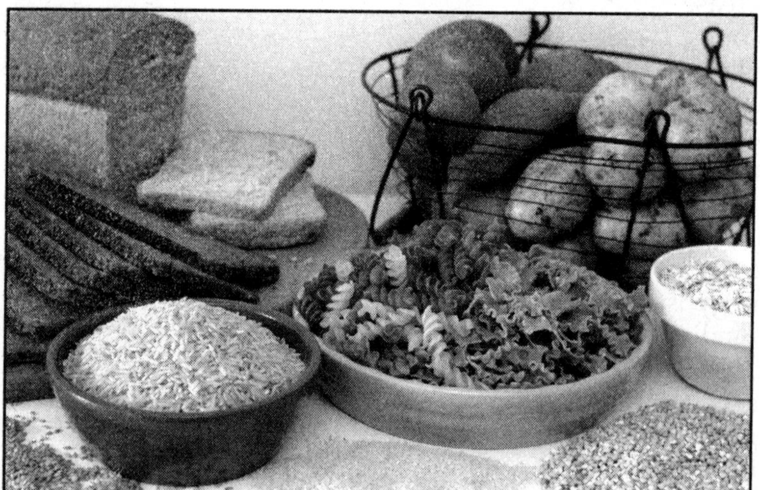

as ideal diet. For example, consuming a larger number of calories in relation to the number of calories spent. The research paper reveals that the food processing industry is busy in encashing the increasing inclination of people towards the food items less in carbohydrates. Such food items contain more of calories. This research paper has also warned that the food products claiming less fat too can prove to be harmful for health. Those who advocate carbohydrates deficient diet, advise to use the glycemic index, too. But following this advice can lead to adverse results. For example, glycemic index of ice-cream is far lower than that of carrot.

It is claimed that food items with less carbohydrates, more fat and more protein reduce weight; while more fat means 60 percent more calories in such food items. Besides, such food products do not mention of any classification pertaining to the kind of fats used in them.

Such types of food items are advertised as a means of weight loss; however, their efficacy is quite doubtful from the viewpoint of health, as the scientific evidences in support of their authenticity is doubtful and negligible. The facts accumulated from the facts pertaining to these food items clearly reveal that if an individual happens to experience some weight loss, it is not due to less consumption of carbohydrates, but calories. But in most of the cases, you can see unprecedented increase in weight because such food items are abundant in calories, fats and proteins. In such cases one has to face the evil consequences. Fat gets accumulated in the vital organs of the body. Not only this, deficient carbohydrates in the body leads to initiation of the ketosis process, which can ultimately harm the kidneys.

Thus, such food items claiming to be deficient in carbohydrates turns out to be a cause of weight gain due to excess amount of fats and proteins. Initially, generation of energy is because of the consumption of fat and protein and an individual feels light. However, at a subsequent stage, the body falls short of carbohydrates due to less intake and body starts consuming the carbohydrates already present in the body. Devouring such a diet can lead to many disease along with heart problems.

□

4

Prepare Diary Notes for Diet and Exercise

Before you set out to undertake a venture of diet control or exercise with a purpose to lose, take a small notebook and annotate the following points:

1. Write the number of times you eat along with the time.
2. Write what all you eat in your diet. Each item should be written with name and quantity.
3. Estimate each morsel.
4. Write the place where you eat – home, office, party or elsewhere.
5. Write whether you feel hungry before you eat or not.

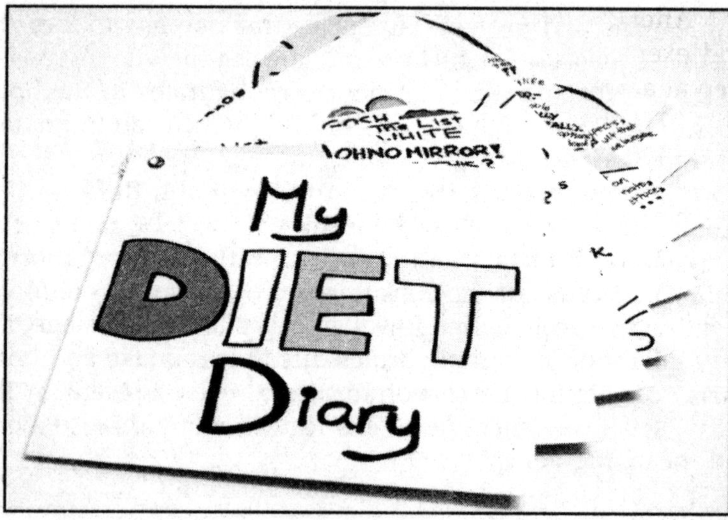

6. Jot down your emotions even if you are tensed or mentally fresh, bored, angry or in a state of guilt at the time of meal.
7. Pen down your total number of physical activities during the day.
8. Check your Weight once a week.

Later, a week or two, analyze the recorded data and compare it with the quality and quantity of the food you had had. This is a way to introspect or self-examination. Therefore, there is no need to mark or rate them as right wrong answers.

1. Do you eat twice, thrice or four times a day?
2. Do you eat spicy food items on regular basis?
3. What is the time interval between two meals?
4. Do you eat to get rid of boredom, guilt or anger?
5. Do you take junk food products having more of fat or calories?
6. How many calories, fat or junk food you consume every day?
7. Are you motivated by hunger to eat or you eat when it is time to eat?
8. Do you undertake any kind of physical activity or exercise?
9. Do you eat while watching television?
10. Do you eat right before going to bed at night?

After this introspection, you can improve upon your eating and exercising habit. It would be more prudent to take one step at a time.

1. Set small realistic targets for yourself which you can implement quite easily. For example, you can add fruits to your diet in order to reduce the food items that have more of calories and fats.
2. Do not aim to reduce your weight by 15 kg a month.
3. The following week, try to reduce the sugary foods from the diet and include more of vegetables.
4. Observe your meal time and decide one timing for your lunch/dinner/snacks.
5. Stay observant as far as calories in the diet are concerned.

□

5

Lose Weight by Powerful Diet

In the present fast-paced way of life, people don't exercise; as a result, obesity engulfs them. If you lack time and unable to exercise but still wish to melt away your increased fat then the alternative you are left with is to change the pattern of your diet to ensure your weight loss.

Morning

Start your day with lemon, honey and water. This would purge the body of all dirt and toxins.

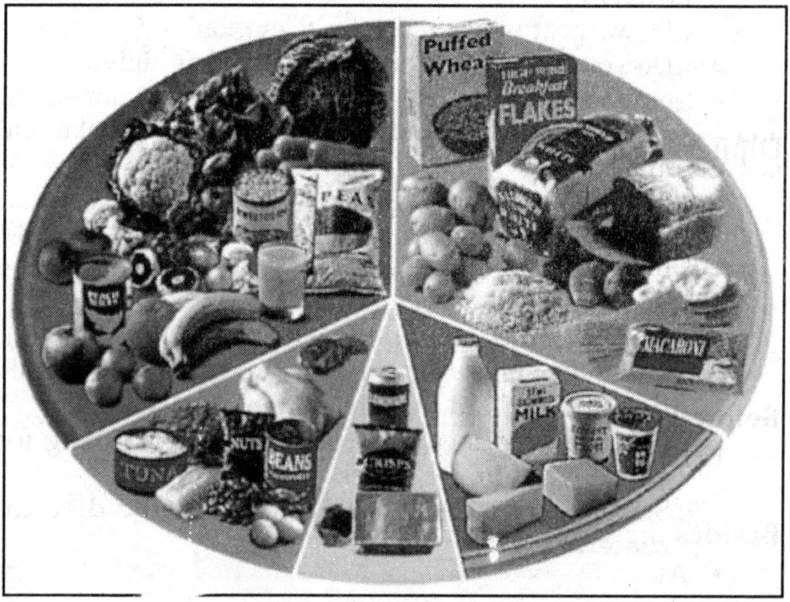

Breakfast

- Omlette of egg-white + 2 slices of brown bread.
- Milk (skimmed) + Cornflakes/oats.
- Fruit salad/Sprouts.
- Poha/Upama.

Before Lunch

Black coffee-It helps to augment metabolism in the body, and you are motivated to do your job.

Lunch

Choose any one of the following:

- Boiled roasted chicken/Soya bean (200 gm) + Brown rice (half plate)/chapatti (1).
- Dal (pulse) + salad + brown rice (half plate), chapatti (1-2).
- Curd (100 gm), it will help in digestion.

Evening

- Eat a sour fruit to eradicate hunger.
- Green tea and two Mary light biscuits.
- Boiled gram.

Dinner

- Boiled soya bean Nutrila, soup + salad.
- Boiled egg white part (3) + vegetable soup.
- Chicken or Tuna salad.
- Boiled dal.
- Dalia.

Before Bed

150-200 ml fatless milk.

Besides the Diet, it is necessary Take Care of

- Avoid heavy dinner. Eat 3-4 hours prior going to bed.

- Drink coconut water, vegetable soup or butter-milk (lassi/mattha) instead of cold drink.
- Drink 2-3 litres of water every day.
- Eat fibrous food, lot of vegetables and fruits to lose weight.
- Limit sugar and sweet intake.
- Never drink water with meals.

□

6

Determination is a Pre-requisite

You gain weight when fat accumulates in the body. Obesity is a serious health condition, which leads to a number of other diseases. Most of the people are obese and not ill. Its onset starts with eating more than required. Each individual requires a definite amount of energy or calorie, which he gets from food. When we intake more calories than the requirement, it gets accumulated in the body as a fat and gradually leads to weight gain.

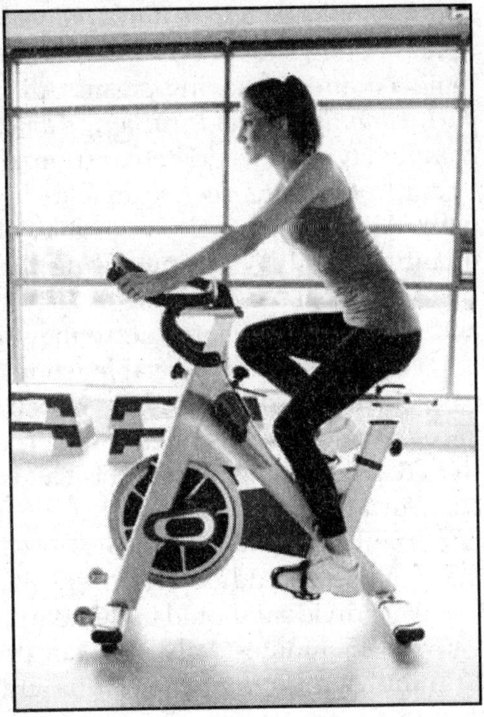

These days, sugary products, sweets, fried and fast foods are in vogue. They are abundant in terms of calories. Besides that most of the people don't burn their calories. Eating more and not exercising are the two primary causes of the obesity. Obesity can be hereditary also. When it is hereditary, an individual cannot reduce his diet in spite of wishing for it. To the contrary, he keeps on eating more and more. Sometimes, obesity can be indicative of other ailments also; like lack of thyroid or growth hormone, excess of steroid hormone and lack of sex hormone. In many cases, children suffer from obesity due to deformity in genes.

Obese people are more likely to acquire diabetes. Due to excess of weight; women are more prone to breast and ovary cancer and men are prone to prostate gland cancer. Besides this, fat people can possibly suffer from colon or rectum cancer too. Over-weight causes complaints of pancreas, stones and arthritis as well. Increasing weight becomes a trouble in respiration process, which is known as 'sleep apnea'. It makes an individual snore during the sleep, and he continues to be listless during daytime. It can have adverse impact on the heart too.

Weight can be reduced with strong will-power. Abstinence from constant and continuous eating should become a regular feature. A diet chart should be got prepared from the doctor and it should be adequately followed by. The quantity of fat (ghee and oil) should be kept to the minimum. Milk should be removed after removing cream. All fried food items, such as *puri, parantha, samosa, kachori, dalmoth, chaat,* etc. should be completely avoided. The consumption of dry fruits, cream, butter, cold drinks, ice-cream and chocolate should be up to a limit. As far as possible, vegetables should be fried in a little quantity of oil. While preparing the food, use of non-stick utensils helps to control the usage of oil and ghee. Frozen oil and ghee are more harmful, so they should be avoided.

Fresh fruits and vegetables should be consumed on daily basis. The gourd, cucumber, radish, lemon and vegetables juices should be consumed more. The non-vegetarian people should avoid eating mutton. Fish and chicken should either be fried in less oil or preferred to be eaten boiled. The most important factor to be taken care while reducing weight is that nothing should be eaten between two meals.

An individual should undertake physical exercise regularly for 30 to 45 minutes daily. You can start the exercise from 5 to 10 minutes a day, which can be gradually increased to 45 minutes in a week. Brisk walking is the simplest of all the exercises. Jogging, skipping, playing hockey, football, badminton, tennis or swimming are good forms of exercises. If you have chest pain or sensitive heart condition, you must consult your doctor before you start your physical exercise regimen.

Medicines in trend for Weight Loss

Recently two new medicines have been invented which help in losing weight. The patients, who are not benefitted by the regular abstinence of food and exercise, can take advantage of these medicines. Besides this, after one has lost weight with the help of these medicines, normally does not gain weight again. One of these medicines is Sibutaramin, which suppresses appetite, and the other is Liptant, which disallows the intestines from digesting fats. These two medicines should only be taken only under the strict supervision of a qualified doctor.

□

7
Lose Weight by Foods

This is needless to say that you need not wander for various recipes in order to lose weight. What one needs is to make a little change in the daily routine and reduce your weight easily. This may sound strange to you, but this remains true to its core.

If we see factually, we will find that the world is struggling against obesity today. Due to this, we find it hard to eat the things we relish and we are forced to undertake dieting. Following list of the food items can actually help you lose weight.

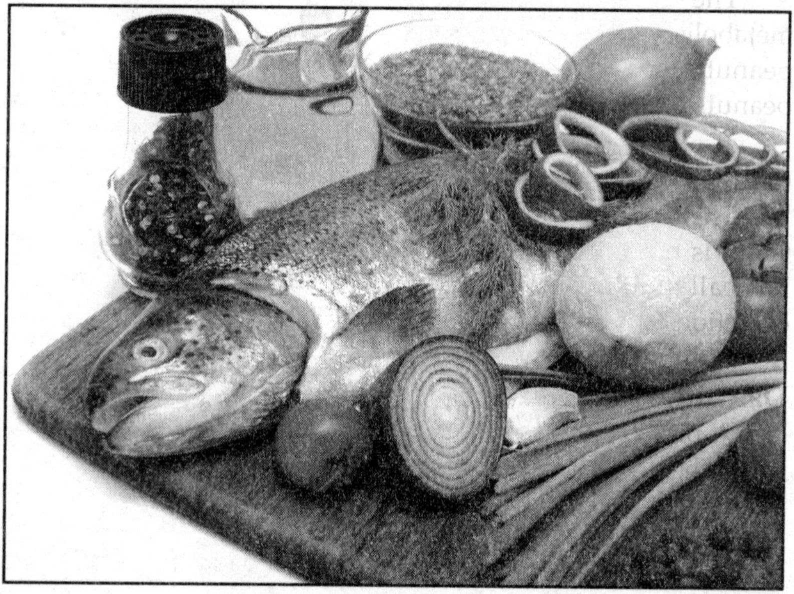

Egg

If you wish to lose weight, eat two eggs regularly. Eggs are equipped with protein and amino acids. This boosts the metabolism of the body, which further helps to slim down. Eating eggs also leads to a jump in cholesterol level, so it is advisable to eat only the white portion.

Oatmeal

Eat oatmeal in the breakfast to mark the beginning of the day well in the morning. It contains high fiber, which makes you feel your stomach full for a longer time. It restricts the rise of blood sugar level. If *dalchini* (Ceylon cinnamon – a type of condiment) is mixed in the oatmeal, weight remains under control.

Garlic

Garlic's constituents help to purge the liver and burn the stored fat in the body.

Peanut

The nutrients found in dry fruits increase the rate of metabolism in our body, and they also provide nutrition. Eating peanut helps to melt away fats. Therefore, eat a handful of peanuts every day.

Chilli

This can be helpful to burn unwanted calories in our body. Chilli is hot in nature and it turns face red when consumed. Basically chillitransforms food into heat that leads to the excretion of a chemical in the form of sweat.

Dalchini (Ceylon Cinnamon)

A pinch of *dalchini* can check your appetite. A number of researches have revealed that the regular use of *dalchini* helps to reduce weight.

□

8

Use Aerobics to Lose Weight

Aerobics is a western style of physical exercise, which has multidimensional objectives. In this technique, the heart rate is gradually increased using different types of exercises and then after bringing to the rapid level, once again it is reduced gradually to bring it to the normal level. The people suffering from heart ailments, high blood pressure, stiff joints and inflexibility need to undertake these exercises only after due consultation with their physical trainers and doctors, else it may prove very harmful.

The objective of aerobics is to regulate the flow of oxygen in the body so that the blood circulation improves with increased heart rate. This leads to a flow of oxygen in the body which results in the production of energy as well as reduction of undesired fat and weight. Its significant ways are as follows:

1. Brisk walking.
2. Jogging.
3. Cycling.
4. Swimming.
5. Walking barefoot on the green grass in the open.
6. Aerobics dance.
7. Skiing.

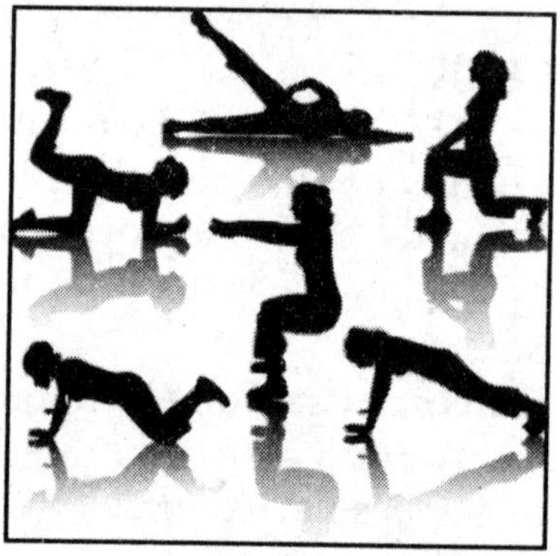

Precautions and Instructions

1. Two people can't be advised for the same kind of

exercises in view of their variance in terms of disposition, physical constitution, capacity, immunity system, types of diseases and other factors. Therefore, one should consult a medical expert before taking up a particular exercise.

2. Aerobics leads to heavy perspiration. The patients, suffering from heart conditions, blood pressure and joint pain need to be more careful as aerobics lead to increased heart rate and pulse rate.
3. These exercises should be undertaken 4-5 days in a week, with an interval of 2-3 days. The exercises can be resumed after this interval.
4. One should get body and blood pressure examined regularly.
5. Ensure that your respiration system gets abundant supply of oxygen; muscles, cells and other organs of the body get constant nutrition and they continue to be active and strong.
6. A healthy body depends on the quantity of blood supplied by the heart. Therefore, adequate and continuous supply of oxygen is necessary for maintaining a healthy heart and regular blood flow which can only be achieved through a regular exercise.
7. Before one sets out to do the aerobics, body should be well prepared for them. (Known as work-up or warm-up). And when aerobics are finished, the body has to be brought back to the prior condition (this process is called cool-down). Both the processes are very important for all.
8. Never stress your body to achieve quick results. Start with light exercises and then gradually increase your rate and time limit over days. When the body gets habitual, go on to the next phase of physical exercise in terms of time, rate and intensity.
9. Always be careful of your body's capability and breathing rate. Avoid excess of anything, else it can lead to more harm than benefit.

□

9
Massage to Lose Weight

Massage is beneficial for the entire body. It helps to excrete toxins from the body with sweat. Massage exercises the whole body. The organs become strong and sturdy; and the laxity of the body is reduced. Unnecessary and excessive fat diminishes from neck, shoulders, arms, stomach, waist, legs, hips, thighs and calves. As a result, the entire body feels light, agile and flexible; besides an increase in mobility of different organs. Massage abates the pain of different organs and joints. Improvised blood circulation increases heart rate and heart's working capacity. Moreover, respiration process becomes uniform and regular.

Massage-Points to Ponder

1. Undertake massage before bathing. Take a bath much before sunrise during summer and at noon in winter; when the sun is at its brightest.
2. Do not massage during monsoon. Because of the moisture in air, one perspires more, hence the body is sticky; therefore, massage is not advisable.
3. The most suitable oil for massage is olive oil. Though its high cost prevents most of us from using it. Mustard oil is a good and a cost effective alternative to olive oil. Both these oils have their own positive attributes. It is still suggested that young children should be massaged with olive oil only; whereas Grown-ups can use mustard oil.

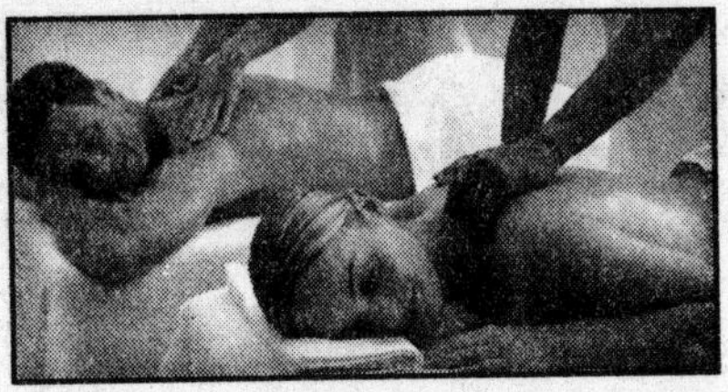

4. Massaging helps to remove body fat, improve blood circulation, cut down muscle fats of the organs and eradicates constipation; and the rectal movement is regularized due to healthier intestines. It helps to improve digestion. Laxity in the body is reduced and the body becomes strong, slim and attractive. As the joints become flexible, they have less pain; the face glows, vision improves and the power of hearing becomes better etc.
5. Always begin massage from down to up. Don't massage forcefully. First apply oil on the body and then massage lightly. Don't strain or apply force.
6. Warm the oil a little before massage, and mix a pinch of salt in it. It helps to assimilate oil into the body more quickly and it seeps down into the muscles. However, keep in mind to massage with the upper layer of the oil only after the salt settles down in the oil.
7. Salted oil enters the body through pores in the skin which excretes sweat. When dirt from the body is removed through massage, the skin becomes luminescent, radiant and soft.
8. Avoid intake of cold drinks before, during or after massage.
9. Always massage in the sun, because the abundant supply of vitamin D helps to pacify number of ailments.
10. Take bath after sitting for almost an hour in the sun. It would help to excrete all toxins with sweat from the body.
11. Bath with lukewarm water. Use good quality soap so that skin doesn't stay greasy. Wipe the body well with a fibrous towel.

□

10

Trivial but Important Points

- Work as per your body's ability and potential. Eat in accordance with the labour you put in.
- The mantra for a healthy life is: eat properly at proper time, work hard and exert enough and take required rest. Whenever these aspects lose balance and coordination with each other, person is likely to invite ailments.
- Do you work yourself but contribute in the tasks outside the house also. Keep your body and mind busy and ensure that you do not waste your time in unnecessary jobs.
- Instead of sitting idle at home, spend your time fruitfully in useful activities.
- Never watch television for long hours. That drains out your energy, affects eyes adversely and weakens them, causes backache as well. Never use the remote; rather move yourself to change channels. Never forget that every set of television is equipped with a button called 'Off'.
- As far as possible, walk down to the nearest bus stand, neighborhood market or shop in order to buy milk, vegetables, fruits and other household articles. Avoid using bicycle, motorcycle, car or other vehicles; they should only be used for a long distance or in emergency.
- Practise yoga every day and do physical exercises. It would keep your body and mind healthy.
- Go for a brisk walk before sunrise till you perspire. It will improve the heart rate, as well as blood circulation. It will lessen joint pain, stabilize respiration process and infuse

oxygen into the body in sufficient quantity and you feel refreshed laced with power, vitality, joy and enthusiasm.

- Use less of sugar, salt and fat in diet. Don't use stale, rotten vegetables or fruits. Always use wheat, gram or bajra flour. The packed flour (atta) is more like *maida* (fine flour) which is very harmful for your health.
- Make more of green and leafy vegetables, seasonal fruits, coconut water, lemon, salad, condiments, spices, pure ghee, mustard oil or corn oil, sunflower oil, soya bean, milk, butter, paneer, buttermilk and other articles important in your daily meal. Keeping in mind your body's condition, as well as kind and level of ailments.
- Don't consume hard drinks like beer, wine, whiskey, country liquor, opium, drugs often for the heck of prestige or fake respect. Excess of fatty and red meat, eggs spoil your health.
- Always prefer home-cooked food over the packed food being sold in market, like pizza, fast foods, chaat, pakoras, fried foods etc.
- Cold drinks, tea, coffee, ice-cream have far more calories so they should be used in a limited quantity and sparingly. Rather, replace all these with fruit juices.

□

11

Morning Walk

The most appropriate time for a brisk walk is prior to sunrise; the air is still fresh, no speeding vehicles around, traffic is rare, the environment is peaceful and pollution free. At this hour of the day, the mind is fresh and body is energetic.

There is comparatively less dirt on roads.

Before you set out for a morning walk, ensure that you:

1. Leave the bed at least two hours before sunrise.
2. Gargle your mouth and drink a glass or two of water as you are habitual or inclined to do.
3. Go for bowel movement (washroom) 15-20 minutes later.
4. Brush teeth after this, and sprinkle cold and fresh water on the eyes.
5. Wear shoes and clothes as per the convenience of walking. Clothes should not be too tight or loose, as it would cause difficulty in breathing. Tight shoes will restrict your fast walk. It would be better if sports shoes are worn.
6. Start walking at a light pace, and then increase the rate with longer steps. If you start walking briskly right from the outset, you will not be able to walk for long and the body will tire out sooner. Maintain equal space in inhalation and exhalation so that you don't get quick breaths. If the path is open and green; take a leisure walk; empty out lungs by deep breathing. Don't take a

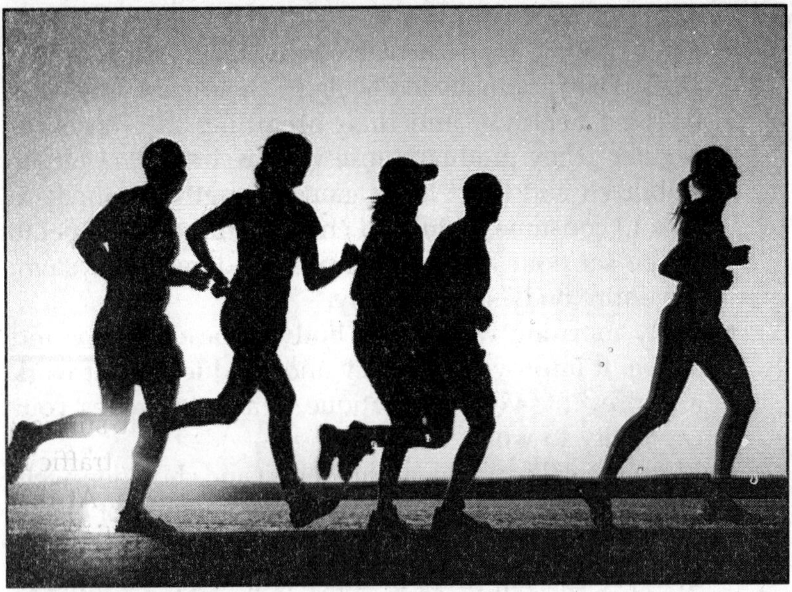

bath soon after you return from the morning walk. Rather wipe the body sweat well and take a rest for a while.

After this, squeeze out a lemon in warm water, add a little black (rock) salt and sugar (diabetic patients can use 1-2 sugar-free tablets) or a spoonful of honey. Obese people should avoid sugar, honey would be a good choice for them. It helps in micturation and excretion of toxins from the body.

Now, take a bath with fresh or warm water as the season demands and get ready for the day.

Morning walk is a pleasant and advantageous physical exercise, so it should form a part of your daily routine. You can avoid it during illness or rough weather. During this time you can take light exercise within the four walls of the house.

Habituate yourself to take dinner early, or 2½ to 3 hours before going to bed. Lying down or sleeping immediately is bad for health and digestion. It takes more time for food to digest. After the night meal, walk a little for a few minutes. Remember, the morning walk should be quick, while that of the night needs to be relaxed.

Advantages of Morning Walk

- Obese people are particularly benefited by the morning walk. They gradually lose weight. Their heart and lungs become healthier and their breathing rate becomes regular. They gradually lose weight, breathing rate is stabilized and heart lungs gains strength. The body is able to consume additional energy, stimulates appetite at the set hour and with improved digestion system, the entire body stays healthy.
- Early morning walk helps body to be energetic and active. It improves efficiency and productivity at work and prevents you from fatique, it also improves your capability to work.
- Morning walk exert legs, arms, chest and shoulders well.
- The brain is supplied with sufficient quantity of blood, which in turn helps ability to think better and focus more. It also improves memory and helps the mind to concentrate more and a person becomes more consistent in efforts.

□

12

Fasting: A Way to Lose Weight

In the Hindu community, much significance has been attached to fasting, it being a part of the religious rituals. This is a meaningful system. As we are inclined to follow the religious rules, each custom and tradition has become a part of our psyche and blood. When fasting is undertaken as an inseparable part of religion, its significance and utility become manifold.

Fasting can be practised in two ways – partial or whole. Under the former system, one or more food items are given up during the day's meal or a meal is skipped. In the latter, a person stays without food and water since morning till night.

Fasting during the period of obesity is still more important. A dietician can be consulted to find out the food items which should be avoided by an obese person. It is advisable to give up such foods forever. Obesity often causes frequent hunger. So an obese person is likely to eat more frequently, as well as eat more. This leaves an adverse impact on his digestive system. It results into digestion-related ailments. Fasting can be observed to avoid such ailments, so that correct measures can be adopted to prevent wrong and excessive eating.

Simple Rules for Fasting

1. Fasting is intended to give rest to the body; it helps excrete toxins, unfavourable and harmful elements from the body and not eat tasty foods.

2. Intake of only those food items, fruits, vegetables and grains which are found in a particular season. Non-seasonal items should be avoided as those products are deprived of nutrients and freshness due to cold storage.
3. On the day of fasting, give up one food item that you eat daily such as salt, sweet, sour, fruit or vegetable. Try to give up the product that you like the most, and without which you feel restless.
4. Eat food only when your mind is at rest and relaxed. Never eat food in a hurry.
5. Never fast during the course of an illness. It can do more harm than good.
6. Don't fast during travel, because it is possible you might have to stay hungry for a longer duration, and it might lead to a decreased sugar level in the body.
7. Chew your food well, don't swallow it. When you chew well, the food is broken down into fine particles, and it is mixed with saliva well. It does not strain your digestive system, and the food can be digested quickly. It would not cause you gastric, sour belches or stomach ache.
8. Don't lie down after meals, nor should you sleep. Rather go for a light walk over 15-20 minutes. If possible, drink a glass of warm water before sleeping.
9. Don't fast during anger, excitement, depression, mental tension or illness etc.

□

13

Calorie-based Food

How many calories does a person need daily, can better be decided in consultation with a dietician or doctor. If you are bored up with a particular food, there are a

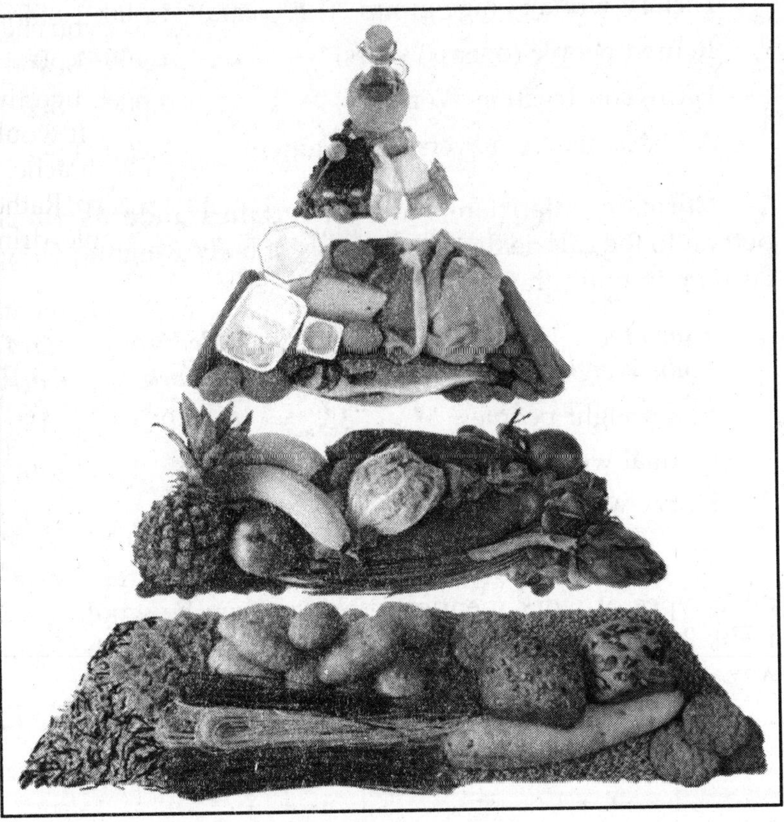

number of other food items that can easily serve as replacement to them. However, this topic should be raised with the dietician or doctor too to obtain necessary instructions; however, no decision should be taken on your own.

Various dieticians have recommended the quantity of calories to be taken by an individual in a twenty-four hour clock and these recommendations are based on the type of work and age of an individual:

Age	*Calories Requirement*
Children younger than 10 years	1,000–1,200
Growing children (until 18 years)	1,400–1,600
Youth (over 18 years)	1,800–2,000
Factory workers (age group 30-40 years)	1,600–1,800
Retired people (over 60 years)	1,400–1,500
Farm/construction Workers	2,000–2,500
Athletes, tennis players, woodcutters	3,000–3,500

Normally, dieticians have set certain standards which pertain to the calorie diet on the basis of body weight (per kg) keeping in mind the total weight and work.

Type of Body Weight	*Sedentary work*	*Medium work*	*Hard work*
Low weight people	35	40	45
Normal weight people	30	35	40
Heavy weight people	20	25	30

For example, if an individual weighs 50 kg; and does all three types of work mentioned above, then he would need 1,750, 2,000 and 2,250-calorie diet respectively. In the same way, calorie-diet can be calculated for other classes.

□

14

Be Strong and Attractive

The easiest and most effective method to prevent weakness of bones is to practise walking on everyday basis. Walking exerts the body in such a way that it keeps the bones strong and they do not decalcify. The bones which are not benefited during the course of walking, become weaker. Decalcification intrudes blood circulation. If you walk daily, your bones remain strong preservation of calcium (which is present in the bones) too is ensured.

If you do not exert yourself daily, you can be inflicted by a terrible disease called osteoporosis. This signifies abnormal loss of bony tissue. This result in fragile porous bones. These types

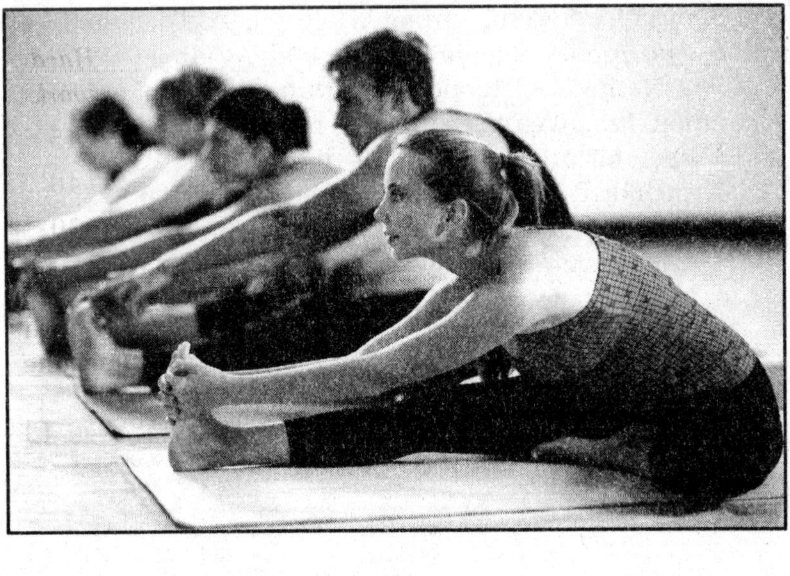

of bones already lack calcium in them. This disease afflicts women more severely, especially after menopause. This disease poses the danger of fragile bones, which can crack. The backbone and waist bones are specifically affected. It makes you bow down and walk, and you appear to be older than your age, because decalcification affects your backbone too.

While walking, keep yourself, your back straight; shoulders parallel to the ground; take every step firmly.

Osteoporosis is a perilous disease. In a country like America, over 2 crore people are afflicted by this disease. There is a sizeable number of 50+ women among the suffering masses. Women are prone to suffer from this disease during the post-menopause phase of life, and the density of bones goes down. As calcium is excreted from the bones, they become hollow. This disease causes change in the shape of bones within the body.

A study report published recently in the *Journal of Orthopaedic Research* has said that the women who continue to work physically even after menopause or 50 years of age, their bones remain strong. Active women in 50-75 age group have denser bones in the spines and arms as compared with inactive women. These women appear younger by 10-15 years too.

Bones also become strong when you walk in sunlight, because it supplies vitamin D to the body.

The National Osteoporosis Foundation, an American institution, has given the following recommendations to men and women for prevention of this disease:

1. Include calcium and vitamin D in your diet.
2. Do physical exercise and walk to decrease weight.
3. Do not smoke, nor should you drink wine.
4. Get the bone density test done in frequent intervals.

□

15

Control Weight, Live Longer!

Physical inactivity and laziness lead to obesity, diabetes, depression, heart disease, arthritis and untimely death. On the other hand, when you walk; oxygen is supplied to the brain and body cells lead to improvement in blood circulation. When sufficient amount of oxygen is supplied to the body, it enhances person's energy and mental agility. Walking also lowers down tension and depression. Thus, mental freshness can be felt by a walk. Walk lowers the level of harmful cholestrol and sugar in the body thus controlling the blood pressure and protecting the heart.

Walking consumes energy or calorie, which helps in prevention and control of obesity and diabetes. Walk strengthens cells of muscles and bones in the body, which protects a person from bone-related ailments. Walking also protects an individual from lung-related diseases and keeps the lungs healthier.

Walking leads to excretion of a chemical called 'interferon', which is very helpful in strengthening immunity system in the body which fights with diseases. Due to this chemical, a person can keep himself safe from a wide range of diseases starting from ordinary cold to malignant cancer. The most important thing about this is that a regular walk can help to protect from untimely death and it begets a long life. Specialists are of the view that everyday and regular walk can help an individual to live longer than the hereditary predetermined time of his death. Many studies have revealed that the people in habit of a daily walk live 10-15 years longer than other people who don't.

All over the world, the walkers have always been amongst the long-living people. Whether it is a Masai tribal in Africa or a Russian tribe in Siberia; whether it is a mountaineer in Peru or a primitive man in New Guinea; tube worker in London or a postman in America – all of them endorse a common characteristic and that is, they all walk. This is precisely the reason why they live longer than other people around them in the same town or country.

Dr. Alexander Chief, a professor of clinical medical department of Harvard Medical School, studied population patterns in different parts of the world, and arrived at a conclusion that active population lives longer than inactive population. He says, "It is evident that one can stay healthy all through life by regular walk. This practice can be adopted at any stage of life and it gives positive results.

In most cases, the causes of obesity are eating more and exercising less. The studies pertaining to life insurance reveal that excessive body weight poses more threats to the heart, and obese people are more prone to untimely death. The same studies have inferred that an individual can live longer by losing weight.

A report was published in the September 2004 issue of a magazine published by the American Medical Association. It says that when old people walk regularly, their mental strength is maintained and the threat of diseases like memory loss is reduced.

□

16

How to Identify Obesity?

Excessive eating leads to a number of diseases. Therefore, let us first find out:

1. What are the symptoms of obesity?
2. There is no doubt about the fact that obesity is a curse.
3. It lowers down the dignity in one's own eyes, he becomes butt of jokes and, in turn, person turns away from being social.

An obese person normally has to face the following situations:

- Muscles of the neck hang down.
- Arms, neck and hands become heavier.
- As the waist increases in size, the belly protrudes out which looks ugly.

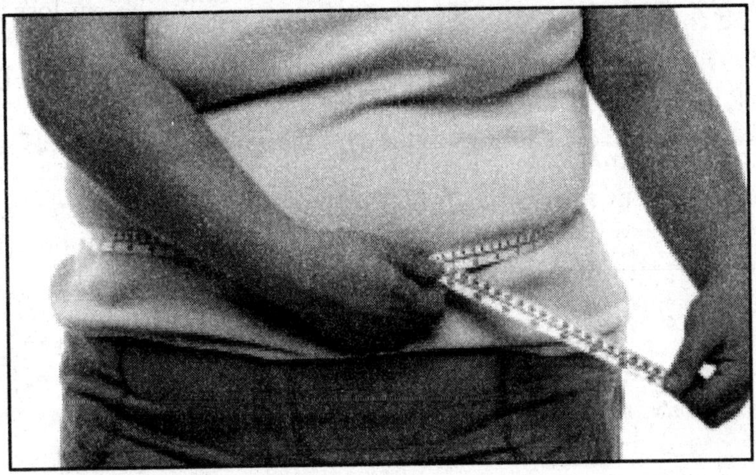

- The shirt becomes tighter at neck, arms, shoulders, chest and stomach.
- The size of trousers increases, and you cannot see your own belt on your waist because the protruding muscles of the stomach hide it.
- As the mass of thighs and calves increases, the trousers become tighter.
- As the mass of muscles increases on legs, socks and shoes do not fit comfortably.
- Even normal walk makes you breathe hard and the body tires out even after a short walk. The situation turns quite painful.
- Post-meal phase leads to sour belches. Gastric problem is faced in the stomach, gas travels in the stomach or gets stuck at one place and may lead to a stomachache.
- There is frequent complaint of diarrhoea or constipation.
- Joints feel pain, bones resonate and get swelled.
- Veins become senseless and the body loses vigour.
- The body tires out after a little work and one gets prone to heavy perspiration.
- Hips become heavier. The way stomach protrudes out and hangs down; the same way, hips protrude towards the back.

There is a simple method to confirm if you are an obese. The fat gets collected under the surface skin. Hold the skin with forefinger and thumb and raise it. If you are not obese, you can lift it by quarter of an inch. However, if you can lift it half an inch, it simply means that the process of obesity has set in and the initial layer of fat has started accumalating under the skin. If the skin can be lifted three quarters of an inch or more, you are certainly inflicted with obesity. This type of situation is a natural warning which should shake you out of slumber, so that you can adopt effective measures to control your weight.

□

17

Should Carbohydrates, Proteins and Fats be given up to Lose Weight?

This is quite a false and misleading notion. In fact, starchy food has been said to be the only form of carbohydrates, which makes up two-third energy deficiency in the body. This energy is the best and cheapest means of obtaining energy. The people who are not aware of the importance and utility of carbohydrates, only they speak of reducing or vanishing it from diet. If we do so, our body will have to depend only on proteins, fats, vitamins and minerals. All these elements together cannot manage the required amount of energy for the body, which

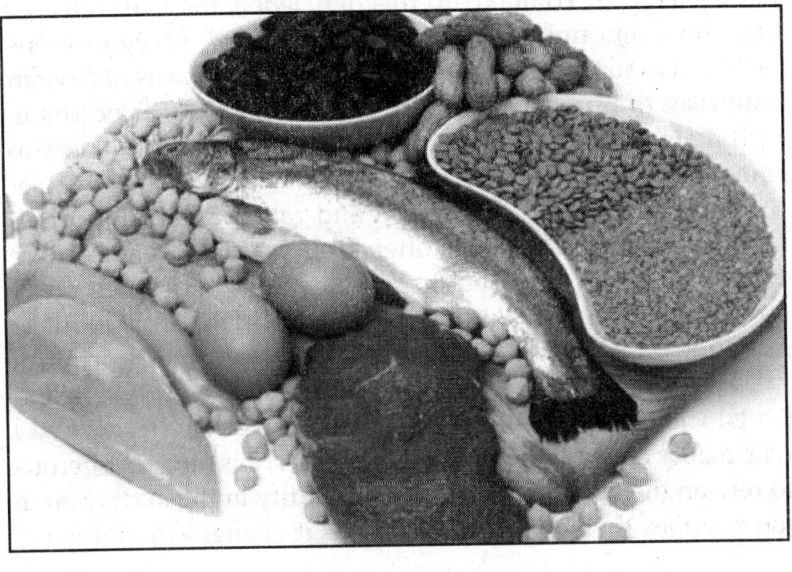

carbohydrates can do alone. Carbohydrates get converted into sugar, glucose and body preserve them in the liver, whenever our body requires them, liver flows carbohydrates into the blood. Therefore, the overweighing people should continue to take carbohydrates in a smaller quantity keeping the state of their digestion and health in mind. This is important so that the digestive system will not have to work excessively in order to generate energy which otherwise can be generated from these carbohydrates. However, it should be borne in the mind that the amount of carbohydrates should match with our daily requirement.

The chief sources of protein are pulses, milk, paneer, curd, buttermilk, fish, egg, meat, soya bean, dry fruits etc. These sources beget us one-third of the required energy. Cereals and grains too give us protein but not in enough amount. If meat is consumed without carbohydrates then the liver changes it first into amino acids then into glucose and fatty acid. Thus, amino group changes into urea that's why it is not beneficial to muscles.

All amino acids should come into the contact with glucose so that they can be used in strengthening muscles. When we physically exert ourselves, our muscles have to work more – they are fagged. To make up this deficiency, the liver releases additional amount of energy into the blood. Oxygen helps the blood to supply glucose to the muscles. The basis of oxygen comprises of pure, clean and fresh air. This process occurs in such a simple and peaceful manner that we hardly come to know about it.

In the same manner, starch and fats play an important role in the body. It has been often seen that we consume more sugar and starch than required by the body. Enzymes break up sugar and starch. Both these are important and useful to make the body strong.

Fat is necessary for proper movement of our bones and joints. Therefore, the role of fat cannot be neglected in the body which does not get accumulated. However, it is more dangerous to rely on the fats for energy which solidify in the body. Starch too supplies the body with energy as it changes into glucose.

In the same manner, the energy obtained from fat is two times more than obtained from any other source; therefore, it is often recommended to limit its consumption in the diet to the minimum.

There is primary need of carbohydrates, proteins, fats, vitamins and minerals etc. for proper nutrition and growth of the body. This proper coordination and balance between above mentioned elements is known as balanced diet.

□

18
Few Exercises in Aerobics

We shall now delineate some exercises under aerobics which can be adopted for weight loss.

Cycling

It is done in two ways – fixed and mobile. The former type of cycling is undertaken within the four walls of the house or gym, and the latter is undertaken on the road; however, the benefits accruing from both are equal. Cycling gives exercise to hips, legs and calves. It removes unwanted muscles from these organs, and they become well-shaped, strong and vigorous. It also increases the heart rate, improves blood circulation and normalises blood pressure. As additional amount of calories is burnt, sugar level goes down in diabetics. Besides, the shoulders, arms and hands also get exerted indirectly. But it does not benefit waist and stomach fat.

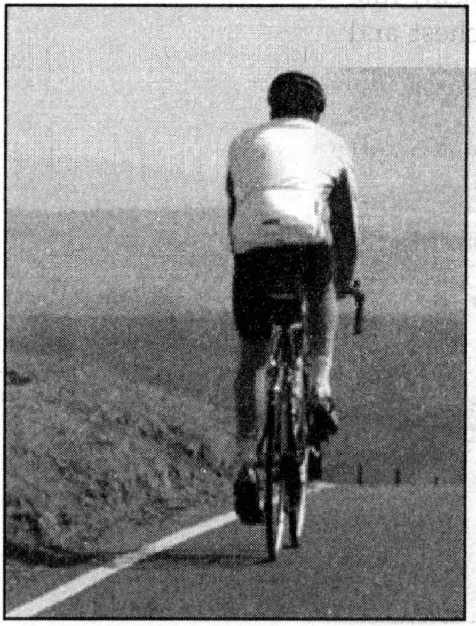

Before going for cycling, you should drink 2-3 glasses of water so that the sweat excreted by this exercise can be easily made up. Water can be had during cycling, but no cold drinks should be taken after cycling is over.

Once you start cycling, start at slow pace and then gradually increase the rate. Keep an eye over your breath. The rate of breathing should not be more than 50 percent of your pulse rate. Towards the end, slow down for a while. Take rest for sometime and allow the breathing to resume to normal rate.

Swimming

Swimming can be done in a swimming pool, river or sea. Those who are not trained in swimming, must learn it only under the watchful eyes of an expert trainer else they should not attempt it. Those who are proficient in swimming, should do it. Swimming is a complete physical exercise by itself, every part of the body gets exercised up. The people suffering from heart ailments, high blood pressure, joint pain in shoulders and legs, asthma, tuberculosis and epilepsy should better avoid swimming, or should practise it only after proper consultation with a medical specialist. Regular swimming helps to diminish obesity, and it makes the body well-shaped, strong, regular and vigorous. It normalizes respiration, blood circulation and heart rate which improves the overall health. It broadens the chest and strengthens shoulders, arms, legs and feet. It also

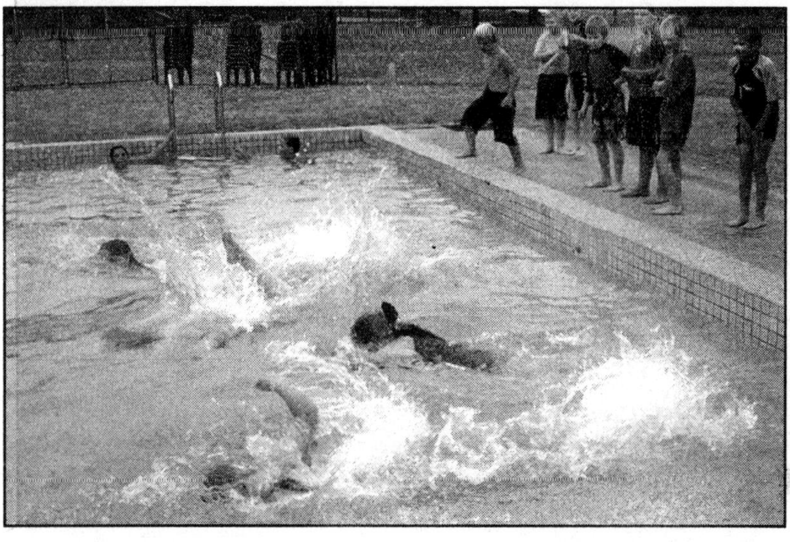

removes loose muscles from the body as muscles become flexible. It improves digestion and the process of excretion of faeces/ urine becomes normal.

Ear plugs should be used before taking into water. Swimming costume should be used for swimming. After swimming, you should change over and then take rest for a while. If you are thirsty, you can drink some liquid. Those who are not well proficient in swimming or are out of practice, should not enter deep water or swift current.

Jogging

Jogging comprises a number of actions, such as slow walking or running, keeping the body mobile, pushing or shaking the body etc. Those who wish to jog should wear comfortable shoes, track suit or half-paint and t-shirt. The shoes and clothes should be well-fitting. They should neither be too tight nor too loose so that they don't pose any problem or difficulty in breathing, walking, running or moving. While jogging, the pressure should be put on hands, feet, arms and shoulders. While running on toes, keep your pace slow else you will not be able to do it over a long distance. When you are breathing swiftly or feeling pain, jogging should be stopped. ☐

19

Lose Weight by Planning

Losing weight might appear to be a hard nut to crack; but the fact is it is not so. Of course it poses some difficulty to those who do not maintain balance and lose the sight. If you have been trying to lose weight over months, yet fail; what you need is not to give up the effort but to make a simple and effective planning.

If you make a plan for weight loss after having given a due thought to this process then you can adopt it in your life and continue all through. Come, let us find out a few of the effective measures to lose weight.

Find out How Much Body Weight You Want to Lose

First ascertain your body mass index or BMI. If needed, take the help of a dietician. Lose weight as per your height. Don't plan to lose more weight in over-enthusiasm.

Fix a Set Timetable

It is not necessary for all people to work out only in the evening. What you have to pay attention is the fact that your time should be regular, that is, it should be at the set hour daily, whether it is in the morning hours or evening hours, it hardly makes any difference.

Undertake Cardio and Weight Training

Cardio and weight exercises are essential for losing weight. Run on the treadmill or road for 45 minutes or undertake cycling.

Don't Take Tension

Only few people are aware that you gain weight by tension. To control tension or stress, undertake yoga, meditation or some hobby for thirty minutes a day and try to be happy at all times.

Play or Do Household Work

To lose weight, sweep the floor, wipe the ground, do gardening or play your favourite sport outside.

Have Liquid

Drink 8-10 glasses of water daily, especially during the course of workout. Besides water, you can also have fruit juice. It will make your skin glow and control your blood pressure as well.

Eat with a Plan

Formulate a good strategy for eating; for example, if you wish to eat some oily or spicy food one day, eat it, but compensate with the suitable physical exercises next day.

Give up Unhealthy Food Habits

You know it quite well that vada pao, ice-cream, milk shake or samosa-pakoras do nothing but increase the level of cholesterol in the body so give them up forever.

Maintain Nutritious Foods in Kitchen

Liberate your kitchen of all packed junk foods and store it with fresh vegetables and fruits. If your kitchen is well-stored with healthy and nutritious foods, you will be able to lose weight quite easily.

□

20

Adopt Easy Methods

Obesity can cause a number of ailments in the body. Initially most of the people do not pay attention to the obesity. They only wake up from the slumber only after obesity has set in. Change in food style is essential to lose weight. There are a number of natural products, whose consumption can help to control weight.

- Intake of wine and milk products should be shunned.
- Boil ginger and lemon in water, and then drink the solution after cooling it.
- Consume at least 750 gm of fruits and vegetables everyday.
- Reduce the consumption of sugar, potato and rice.

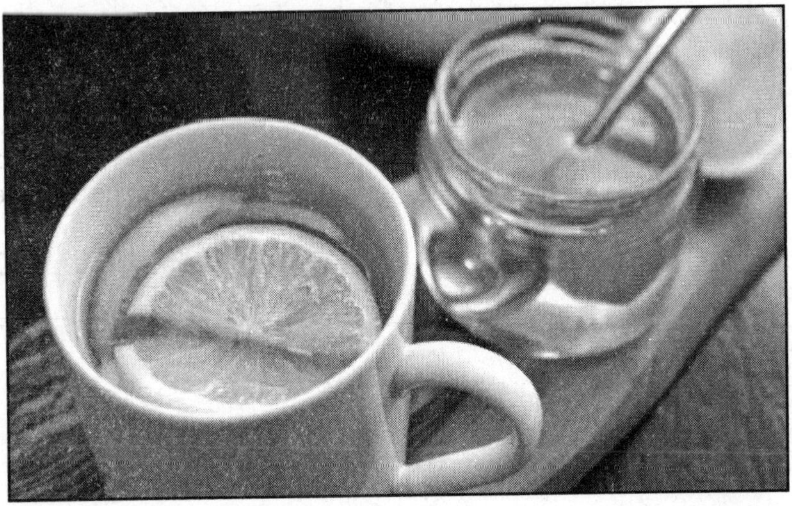

- Chapattis made from a mixture of wheat, soya bean and gram are more beneficial than those made only from wheat flour.
- Include fibrous foods in your daily diet. Green vegetables and fruits have abundant amount of fibre in them.
- Don't eat peeled up fruits. Don't remove potato peal.
- Mix a spoonful of honey and half a spoonful of lemon juice in warm water. Its consumption helps in removing extra fat from the body. It should be taken thrice a day.
- Cabbage has an attribute of reducing fat. It strengthens metabolism in the body.
- Mix a spoonful of *pudina* (mint) in two spoonfuls of honey. It helps to control obesity.
- Drinking of 250 gm of tomato soup in the morning hours over 2-3 months helps to lose fat in the body.
- Carrot juice is useful in controlling obesity. Drink 300 gm of carrot juice at any time of the day.
- Drink at least 10 glassfuls of water during the day.
- Use foods having less calorie value while preparing meal.
- Include lemon, lettuce, grapes, apple, melon, jamun, papaya, mango, orange, tomato, watermelon, strawberry etc. in your diet.
- Consume more of cabbage, cauliflower, broccoli, onion, radish, spinach, turnip, garlic, etc.
- Limit the use of salt in your diet.

□

21

Do Pole Dance and Lose Weight

You might have got bored with the prevalent methods of weight loss – the same monotonous morning jogging and skipping. If this is the case, it is the right time to do something new. This should be something which should help you lose weight as well as give you some recreation. One such method is pole dance. This begets you both – excitement of dancing and opportunity to lose weight. You must have seen pole dance performances on television or internet. You might not have imagined then that this can help you lose weight. Pole dance helps to melt away additional fat from the body which leads to an agile, vigorous and fit you.

Let us find out the benefits of pole dance.

Keeps the Heart Healthy

Pole dance is a good exercise for the heart. Everyday one hour of this dance and that too regularly helps you burn 200-450 calories. Its greatest benefit is that it is not an ordinary physical exercise that you see around you. It recreates you too. You don't have to motivate yourself daily for doing this. So,

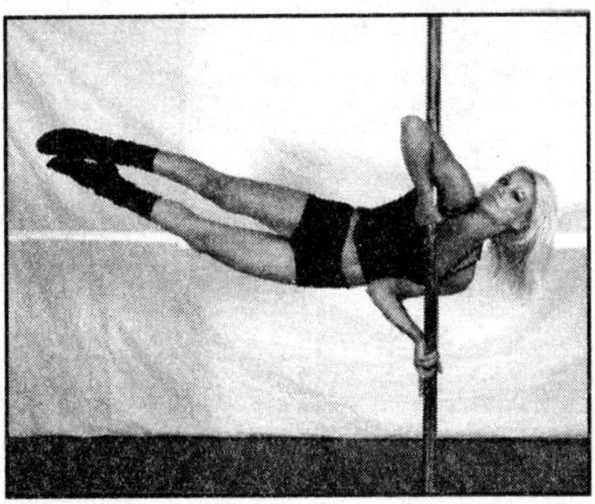

you can better say that have the cake and eat it too. While doing it, you will hardly realize the completion of one hour.

Burns Fat

Not only particular organs get exercised up with Pole Dance but whole body also. It enhances the activities of hands and feet. Due to irregular lifesytle fat gets accumalated in the body and results in a shapeless body. However, regular routine of pole dance shapes and tones your muscles. When you gain weight, you often have heavier thighs and hips. Such type of fat melts away in pole dance and you gradually have stronger muscles.

Cultivates Self-confidence

Pole dance helps you to keep fit as well as inculcate self-confidence because it makes you feel good. Other physical exercises certainly shape your body and tone your muscles up but you cannot enjoy them all. Pole dance makes you feel good within you. Pole dance is liked by all, especially womens. It cultivates self-confidence in them.

While undertaking pole dance, the following points must be kept in your mind:

- If you feel something scary about the pole dance class, take somebody along with you.
- Wear those clothes for pole dance which can help you dance well and freely. Avoid applying any kind of cream or oil on hands; it can make your hand slippery while holding the pole.
- No experience is needed to do pole dance. This can be learnt only by practice. With time, you will learn it well.

□

22

Lose Weight by Yoga

The nature bestows upon man a balanced and a well-shaped body but he spoils its shape with his wrong lifestyle, bad habits and improper and irregular eating habits. In scientific terms, by obesity is meant more body weight in relation to height. In the present scenario, this ailment is engulfing the world like never before.

The most important cause of obesity is that we do not undertake much physical work in relation to the food we eat. The energy produced in the body remains unburnt within the body due to lack of physical work and this energy gets collected in the form of fat.

Fat gets collected first on hips and waist. When the belly hangs, muscles lose their tone. Loose muscles hanging on hands

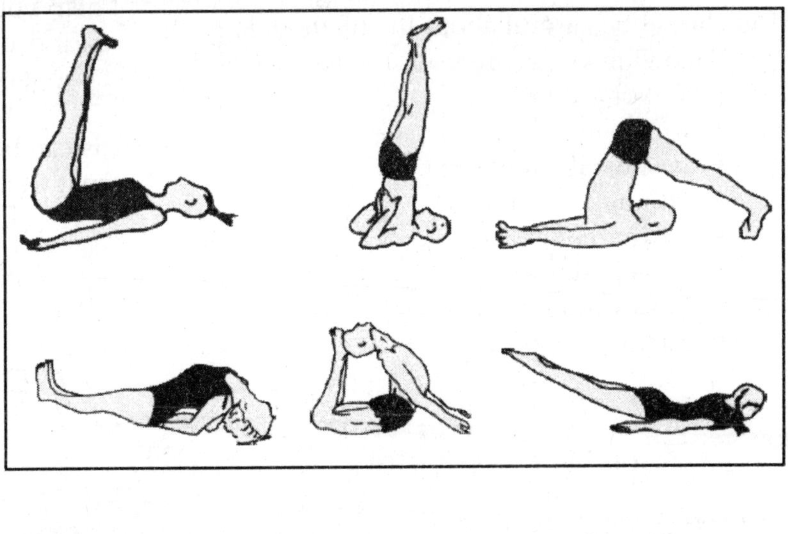

and thighs are indicators of obesity. Obese people suffer from constipation; there is every possibility of their becoming victims of diabetes, high blood pressure, heart disease, joint pain, arthritis and knee pain.

Take a brisk walk for at least three km a day. Besides, running, swimming, playing games and cycling too are advantageous. Yoga is considered to be the most apt method as it helps both mind and body to stay healthy. Kapalbhati pranayama should be done for 15 minutes everyday.

You should observe your diet along with yoga. Green leafy vegetables, seasonal fruits and fruit juice are useful. The diet should comprise of salad, soup, butter milk and curd, which help in digestion. Eating fruits after meals helps in digestion, such as papaya, guava.

You should only eat if hungry and as per your appetite. Reduce the use of sugar, salt, sweets, ghee and oil for a better results. Sitting in Vajrasana posture for 5-10 minutes after meals helps in improving the digestive system.

While doing yoga, you should focus your mind and breath to the yoga and accompanying activities. Each activity should be performed with long and deep breath. It helps in contraction and expansion of different body organs as a result benifitting all the organs.

Taking training from a trained and professional yoga teacher helps to a great extent. Doing it at home also helps but you should be careful about the methodology.

Following yogas are useful to lose weight:

- Trikonasana.
- Konasana.
- Pashu vishramasana.
- Uttanapadasana.
- Ardha-halasana.
- Padavrittasana.
- Pavan muktasana.
- Surya Namaskar.

□

23

How Children can Lose Weight?

Obesity is an atrocious problem which the world is facing, and it has made people susceptible to serious problems. Due to modern lifestyle, children have become more susceptible to obesity as compared to the previous times. Obesity in children has resulted in diseases like diabetes. Modern lifestyle, conjoined with modern technology has multiplied the problem of obesity in children. If children exercise regularly, they can keep their weight under control easily. Now the pertinent question is to ascertain the exercises which help children to reduce and control weight and what can be the other benefits of these exercises.

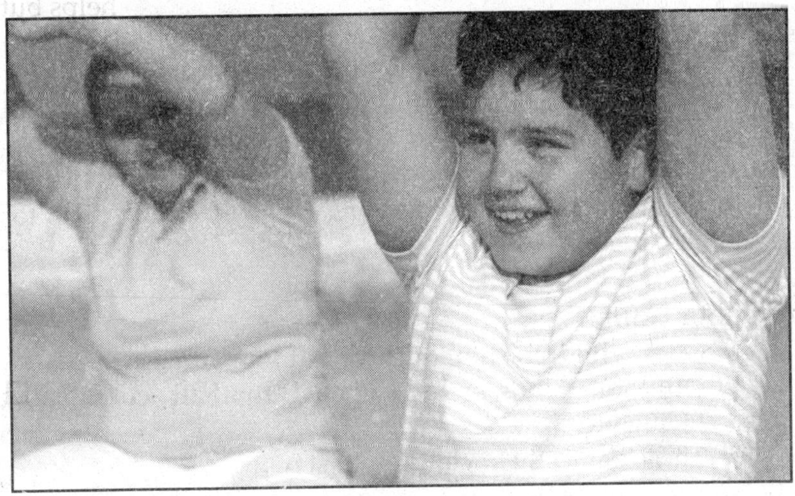

Come, let us find out the exercises for children that can help them lose and control body weight.

Swimming

- Generally, children love playing in water. If children swim for recreation, it would be helpful in maintaining their health too. Children derive a hoard of benefits from swimming.
- Swimming can help children not only in losing weight, but also in strengthening their muscles and body.
- Swimming allows children to undertake the physical exercise of the entire body. Swimming everyday can turn children into fit and fine individual.

Cycling

- Children love to do cycling and when the same cycle helps them keep fit, they will certainly love to mount on it and enjoy themselves.
- 30-minute cycling a day keeps children fit and helps them reduce their weight.
- The children, who are yet to learn cycling can take to a stationary bicycle. It will help them have physical exercise as well as lose extra body fat easily.

Skating

- Children suffering from obesity should go for skating. The more time they devote to skating, the better physical exercise they will have, the fitter they will become.
- Children can compete with their friends in skating. It will give them physical exercise while helping them to lose weight.

Outdoor Games

- Obese children should go for outdoor games.
- Outdoor games include cricket, football, volleyball, racing etc.
- These games help children to stay fit.

- Children can easily lose weight by playing outdoor games, because it exercises their whole body.

Jogging

- Children should be sent for jogging to lose weight.
- If your child is not inclined to do physical exercises, then send him out for a walk or make him busy in a game in which he can jog too.
- Jogging is not strenuous yet it makes a child healthier.

□

24

Care in Eating

Obesity enhances the possibility of a number of diseases. Therefore, it is essential that you should be wary of obesity and keep it under control. Besides exercises, you should take care of your diet too. Taking some precautions help you eradicate obesity.

Don't Drink Water after Meals

Often people drink a lot of water after meals, which is not

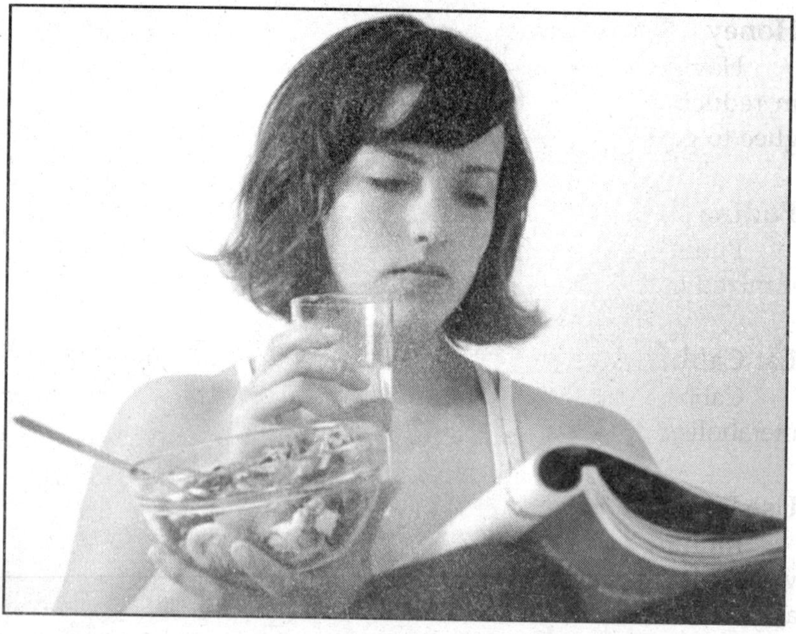

advisable. Water should be consumed only half an hour after lunch. It does not allow your waist and stomach to inflate, and helps to control obesity too.

Use Green Leafy Vegetables

Your diet should predominantly comprise of green leafy vegetables, leaves and salad. Their quantity should be more than chapatti and rice. It will not allow fat to accumulate in the body.

Fast for Benefits

If possible, observe fast once a week and during this time, consume only milk and fruits. It will help you improve your digestion.

Eat Chapatti of Barley-Gram

Replace your wheat flour chapatti with barley-gram (jau-chana) flour chapatti. It will not only slim down your waist and stomach but the entire body also.

Honey

Having two spoonfuls of honey in warm water too helps in reducing obesity. Don't stop the intake of milk and pure ghee to get slimmer, it can make you weak.

Pudina (Mint)

Pudina or mint is very useful in slimming down. Having it mixed in honey helps to reduce obesity.

Eat Cabbage

Cabbage has traits of losing fat and it strengthens the body metabolism.

Use Fibrous Vegetables

Include more of fibrous foods in your diet. Green vegetables and fruits have lots of fibres so eat them as much as you can.

Drink More Water

Drink more of water. It helps in increasing metabolism process in the body. This in turn will help burn more calories, ultimately helping in fat loss.

Fibrous Foods

Eat foods which have fibre like almond, beans, popcorn and brown rice. They help in reducing body fat.

Don't Give Up Eating

Have your breakfast, lunch and dinner on time. Don't skip meals at any time because it makes you eat more in the next meal; therefore, eat at the scheduled time.

□

25

Mistakes that Lead to Weight Gain

Eat Hurriedly

Eating in a hurry is a wrong eating practice. If you do this, your nervous system doesn't get time to convey to your brain that the work of eating is over. Therefore, when you eat in a hurry, you don't feel full enough. Chew every morsel of food well and enjoy eating it. It will beget you contentment even if you eat little and you will not feel like eating again and again.

Give Up Breakfast

Often people entertain a false notion that giving up morning breakfast will help them reduce their weight. This is factually wrong. Those who give up breakfast gain weight more quickly than those who take it. When we wake up in the morning, we have already fasted for close to eight hours; it is at this hour that we need sufficient quantity of calories to work for the whole day. If you skip breakfast, you may not feel yourself, but if you happen to eat

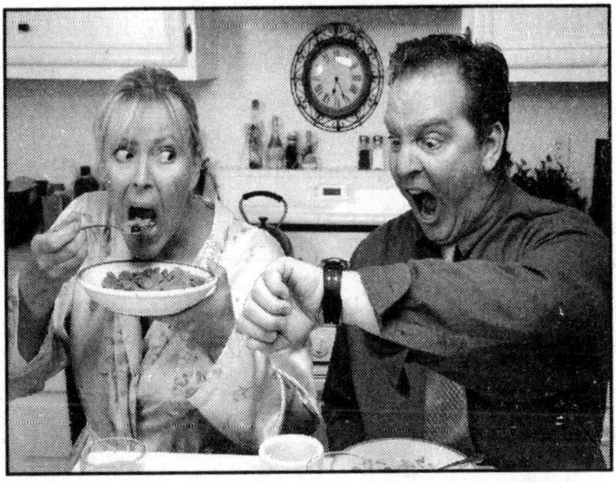

intermittently in the form of biscuits or wafers, it can only make you gain weight. Therefore, having breakfast is essential.

Binge Eating

Some people are not able to estimate their appetite well. When they go to a restaurant for meals, they order for more dishes than they can eat; and argue in favour of not wasting food, they eat more than necessary. In the same manner, some women may not have a proper idea of the food items they cook; which results in their cooking more food than is required in the family. This remains a prime cause of their weight gain. Use smaller dishes while eating. It will make your food look more and you will feel as if you have eaten more.

Selection of Wrong Items

Some people think that if they take only salad or soup in meals, it would not affect their weight adversely; however, dressing on salad or butter in soup are enough to make up the deficient calories. Can you lose weight this way? Therefore, take salad without dressing and never put butter in soup.

Tit-bit Eating

Some people take to light eating oftentimes just to kill boredom but this light food makes their bodies heavy. Such type of eating habit is called eating amnesia. Such people are inclined to keep something in their mouths whenever they open the refrigerator, or they just extend their hands for chocolate or sweets at any time of day. Some people eat wafers or biscuits while watching television or reading a book. It is hard to control such a habit. Therefore, if you have such type of problem then keep fruits near you while watching television or reading a book; or have herbal tea. Always have a bottle of water handy with you and whenever you feel like eating something, go for the bottle. Chewing gum can be a right solution for this type of tendency.

□

26

Lose Weight During Thyroid

The thyroid gland in our body has been assigned the duty of controlling metabolism. When this gland does not work efficiently, it can create a number of health problems. Hyperthyroidism is one such condition. In this condition, the thyroid gland starts to producing more thyroid than necessary; and on the other hand, in hypothyroidism, this gland produces less amount of thyroid. Both these conditions require different types of treatments. Hyperthyroidism leads to decreased weight, while hypothyroidism leads to increased weight. It is not easy to control weight during this illness.

Therefore, let us find out how can we keep the body weight under control during thyroidism.

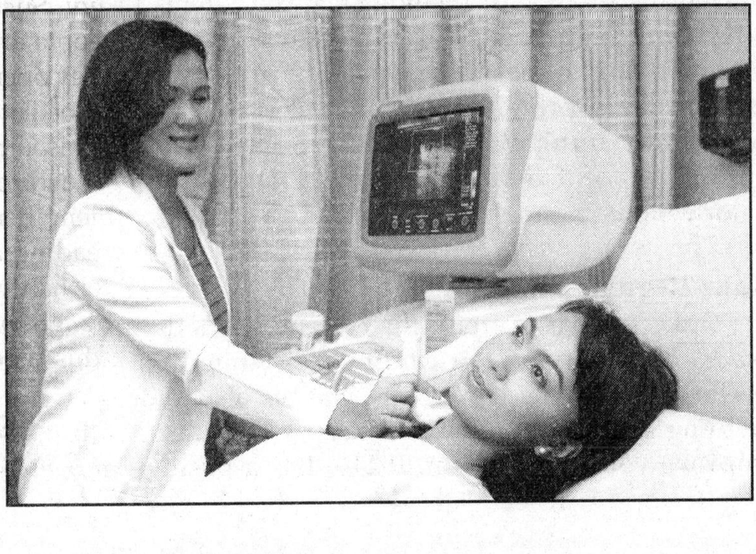

Medical Check up

The first thing is to get medically examined, to ascertain the type of thyroid; whether it is underactive thyroid or overactive thyroid. After the examination reports, doctor will advise you further course of action. The doctor will also examine if you have any hard lump or swelling on the neck/ throat. If there is, he will examine its type and if it is related with thyroid. Necessary examination help him to arrive at a definite viewpoint about the actions in terms of daily routine and treatment that you can take up to keep your weight under control.

Take Medicines on Time

Pay attention to the fact that medicine to cure thyroid should be taken timely and regularly. Some medicines prescribed for underactive thyroid have impact over metabolism too, which help to reduce weight. After transplant surgery, thyroid gland starts functioning better and this helps in keeping the body weight under control.

Eat Good

If you wish to attain a positive outcome as far as your body weight is concerned then be careful about your diet during the treatment. Include such food items in your diet which will keep your digestion system healthy. You should also take care to include vegetables, fruits and low-fat dairy products and protein foods in your diet. Ensure that you never stay hungry. Whenever you feel hungry, prefer vegetables and fruits. Keep away from chips and high calorie foods.

Take Regular Exercise

Take regular exercise for 30 minutes daily, five days a week. If you wish, you can go for swimming, jogging or cycling. Besides these exercises, you can also undergo weight training exercises, which will keep your heart healthy and improve your metabolism. It also has a positive impact on your thyroid. Doing exercise helps to keep your body fit as well as control weight.

Follow Doctor's Advice

Keep consulting your doctor. Don't be negligent on this aspect. The doctor can examine the level of your thyroid on regular basis and advise you a better course of treatment and diet.

□

27

Seven Rules to Avoid Weight Gain

We often wonder how we can control our desire to eat? Or how can we make it possible to eat what we desire and still keep our body weight under control? For this, you have to follow seven simple rules given under:

1. Separate Eating from Television

If much of your time is spent in eating, napping and changing television channels, you are sure to gain weight. For this, first choose nutritious and light foods; take only as much as is required by you in your plate. Always pay attention to the quantity and the quality of what you are eating.

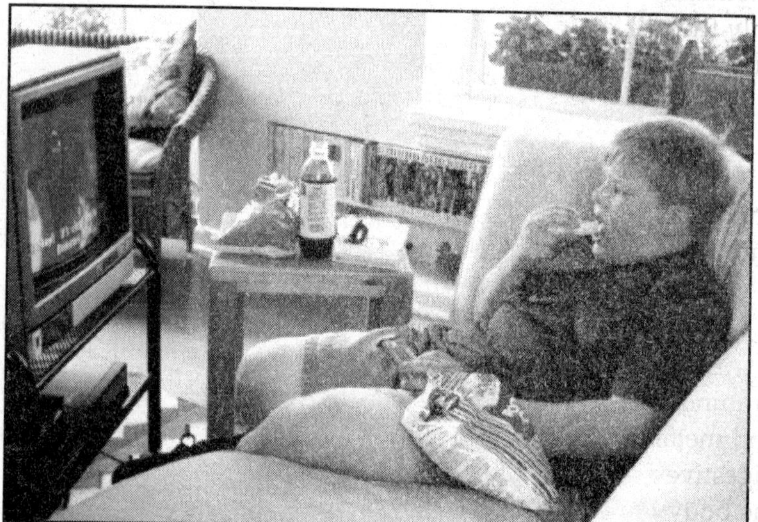

2. Don't Skip Meals before Party

If you are scheduled to attend a party in the evening, don't starve yourself through the day. If you keep eating at the right intervals, you will save yourself from eating excessively. We have an inbuilt body clock and metabolism runs according to the set cycle. If you eat on the scheduled time, you will not feel hungry excessively and you will be able to turn away from unreasonable eating.

3. Break for Deep Breathing

Do you start eating when you are angry, tired, bored up or tense? Before you undergo any such emotions, just cool your mind down and think over it. Breathe deeply and long for number of times. It will bring down your rage and stress. You will be able to distinguish between real hunger and sentimental hunger. Eat when you have genuine hunger.

4. Don't Deviate

This remains a fact that even a determined and resolute person can deviate from daily routine and eat some thing like a fruit in between the meals. But make sure to return to your fixed daily routine as soon as possible, taking that instance as only the exception. Never think that once you have violated a rule, you can violate it everytime.

5. Exercise without Pretence

Include physical exercise in your daily routine. Make it an important part of your daily life. Put it as a reminder for yourself and get on it like any other important task of the day.

6. Eat Several Times, Eat in Limit

Eat six to eight times a day, but eat in less quantity. Keep in mind that your body requires only few calories for energy and metabolism. When you eat more at one go, it strains your digestive system and the remaining calories get deposited in the body in the form of fat.

7. Share with Others

Sharing your food with others is a good habit. It gives you a better taste and your share of food goes down which reduces the number of calories being supplied to the body. That means that you can eat what you desire and still keep fit. The only thing to look for is, its quantity.

□

28

Five Foods to Lose Weight

1. Salad

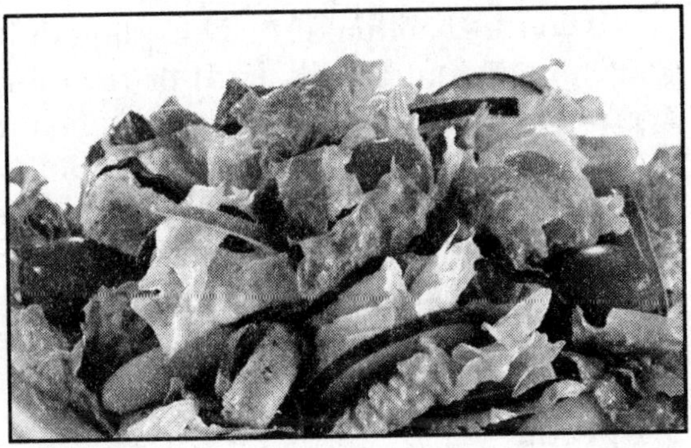

Your morning and evening meals should necessarily have a reserved place for salad. If you wish to have less of calories and more of fibres, then salad is the better option for you.

The raw vegetables and fruits used for salad contain antioxidants, natural enzymes and fibres which help to control cholesterol as well as improve digestion of food in the body. They also help in keeping your body weight under control. If you wish to lose weight, you must eat a large bowl of green salad daily.

2. Whole Dals or Pulses

Whole or unpeeled dals or pulses have an abundant amount of protein. Pulses also have folic acid, vitamin A and vitamin B. Their daily consumption helps to reduce the level of cholesterol in the body, consequently controlling your body weight.

3. Yellow and Citric Fruits

Of all fruits, citric fruits have better qualities. Yellow and orange coloured fruits have beta keratin and antioxidants. Sour fruits are primary sources of vitamin C, calcium, minerals and fibres etc. which are useful for body's growth. Pectin is present in lemon, which melts the fat collected in the body. It also slows down the digestive process which pacifies appetite.

Citric fruits are good for the people suffering from diabetes, cancer, anaemia, cataract, asthma, kidney stone etc. Consumption of these fruits increases immunity system of our body also.

4. Liquids

If you are habituated of taking liquids before or after meals, you can take buttermilk, curd or fruit juice. These fluids are good for your body. Lemon juice is helpful in losing weight, protecting teeth, controlling fever and blood sugar. Buttermilk is deficient in fat and can be taken after meals. Coconut water has abundant amount of potassium which controls blood pressure as well as increases immunity system of the body. It also has lower amount of carbohydrates, sugar and fat.

5. Sprouts

When grains are sprouted their nutrient value doubles. Gram (chana), lentil (moong), soya bean, peas, etc. can be sprouted to eat. Sprouted grains can also be consumed together with soup or salad.

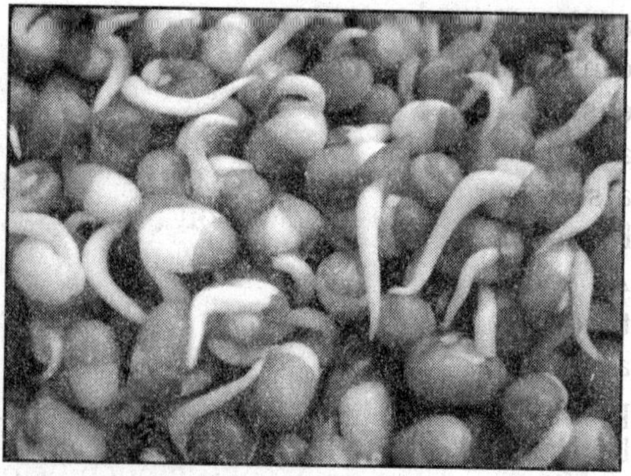

□

29
Drink Soup to Lose Weight

We think of soup only when we fall ill. We simply ignore the fact that soup can play a vital role in keeping us fit.

Generally

When we speak of continental dinner, we start our meals with soup as a starter. The thought behind this is the fact that soup stimulates the appetite and then you can enjoy your dinner well enough. The fact also remains the same that it is good for health. If you include soup in your daily diet, it keeps you fit. At the same time, you develop a good appetite.

Soup is also taken as a medicine. If you are having stomachache or facing problems in chewing food doctors often advise soup as light food. The positive aspect of soup is that it can be digested easily. In addition to it, it also controls blood pressure. As soup has all types of minerals and vitamins, it protects our body from dehydration. According to a report, soup can

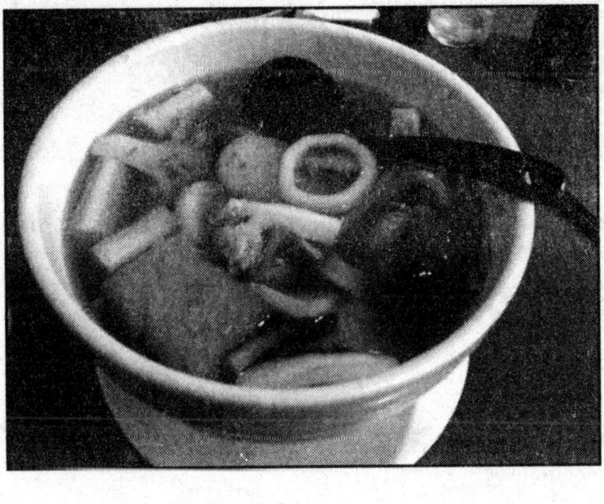

bring down the danger of breast cancer. If you are suffering from cold or fever, you can be benefited by chicken or vegetable soup.

More Fibres

Children often avoid vegetables, especially green and leafy vegetables. To ensure nutrition in children, it is essential that they get adequate amount of protein and minerals. Soup is very good for health as it contains a lot of fibres. The best thing about this is that number of vegetables can be used together, such as carrot, cabbage, cauliflower, tomato, beans and spinach. All these have a lot of fibres in them. Besides, you can bring about a change in its taste by introducing different types of vegetables on different occasions. It will give you different tastes at different times while supplying the body with adequate amount of fibres.

Effective in Reducing Weight

The people who desire to lose weight, they ought to know that soup is effective for this purpose. Specialists opine that cauliflower soup is good to reduce weight. Its greatest advantage is that it does not weaken your body while dieting. It supplies the body with essential minerals and nutrients. Most of the dieticians include soup in their diet plans and health charts because it serves as calorie or energy source instead of fat. It doesn't make you weak and keep you fit.

Enhances Beauty

Together with health and supply of fibres, soup is also helpful to enhance beauty in women. Soup enhances and strengthens the immunity system. It prevents wrinkles and spots. Your body gets a balanced diet in the form of soup. As a result skin glows resplendently.

□

30

Daily Routine and Weight Loss

In the recent years, people have grown conscious about increasing obesity. Fit people wish not to gain weight while the obese people somehow wish to lose weight. Let us see how we can achieve these objectives.

Don't Skip Any Meal

If you wish to lose weight, the foremost thing to do is not to skip any meal. Eat three meals and two refreshments during the course of a day. If you skip a meal, you are bound to eat more in the next meal.

Pay Attention to Breakfast

Some people skip breakfast thinking it might help lose weight. However, the researches reveal that if you have breakfast regularly, you lose weight in a long period of time. Don't eat the same thing in breakfast or morning meals. Keep changing food items. You can take a whole lot of things like *dalia* with milk, veg sandwich, poha or upama.

Have Dinner Early

The day meals should be nutritious while the dinner should be light. It should be eaten by 8 o'clock in the evening. If it is not possible, eat at least two hours before going to bed. Don't eat things like dals, curd, rajma (kidney bean), rice etc. in dinner as they are hard to digest. If you keep awake late into the night, you can feel hungry. At that time you can take fruits or salad. In fact, the digestive process slows down during the night, so it takes longer to digest food at night.

Be Aware of the Quantity

Pay attention to the quantity of food; that is, it is better to have a bowl of boiled gram than to have a couple of biscuits because both of them have similar amounts of calories. You can also take beans, salad, *dhokla*, paneer (toned milk), gram etc.

Cut Down on Salt

Don't add salt from above. Of course, nutritious food does not mean tasteless food. Traditional condiments and spices help to augment the taste and tickle taste buds; they also contain micro-nutrients, fibres and antioxidants. Only thing needs to be taken care of is that not much oil should be used to fry them.

Whole and Unpeeled Items are Better

Don't sieve flour to make chapattis. Mixing gram flour with wheat flour helps in better digestion. You can eat wheat or barley flour (without sieving), brown bread, dalia, corn or wheat flakes, brown rice and pulses etc. Sprouted grains and pulses are abundant in vitamins, minerals, proteins and fibres. □

31
Dietary Rules

- Eat food slowly. Take in small morsels and chew each of them well.
- When you have finished the food served for the first time, wait for at least 15 minutes to decide whether you really need more food. Your apostate (the system in the brain that controls appetite) will by then feel satisfied and you will feel like eating more food.
- Decide upon the place of eating in the house. If you don't do it, maybe you will like to eat something in every room of the house. If your eating place or room is definite, your habit of eating all the time will be controlled.
- Don't sit at the dining table long after you have finished eating. Besides, spend less time in kitchen or other such part of the house where you feel like eating.
- While eating, don't place additional food items on the dining table. If you have more food items, you will feel like taking second and third time also. Place food items in such a way that they are easily visible.
- Never go to the market hungry. If you do so, you will be motivated to eat junk food in the market. Besides, don't form a habit of eating while watching television or reading a book. When your attention is not focussed on eating, you can eat more than required.
- Before the time of vacation/weekend, start physical exercise regularly in order to lose weight in advance. If

you think you can postpone this work for the free time, then it will not be an easy task to accomplish it.

- Avoid fried items. Such foods have lots of fat, which oversupplies the body with calories.
- Have soups. In addition, include food items which require more chewing. The things you can chew for longer, give more satisfaction.
- Eat salad before the main meals. It will reduce your appetite and you will not be able to have food containing more fat or calories.
- Alcohol contains 7 calories per gm; so drinking alcohol can have adverse effect on the plan to lose weight. If you are serious about losing weight, give liquor up and drink lemon water regularly.

□

32

New Diet Plan to Lose Weight

Obesity has become a common problem with people. Lot of methods and tricks are being applied to lose weight and keep fit; right from keeping hungry to excessive workout. Such people simply forget that not taking proper care of their diet, they are only putting their health at risk. If some diet plan can be used to stay healthy, why will you need to stay hungry?

DSH Diet

DSH is quite popular at the international level. It means

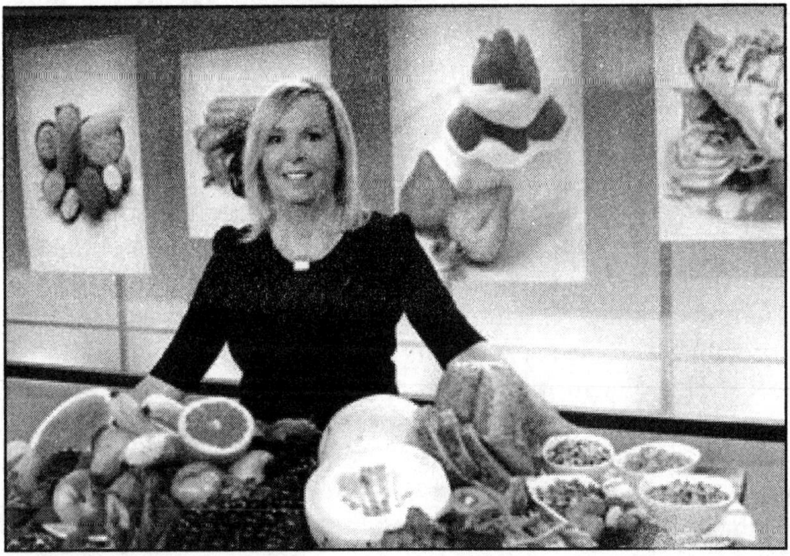

'dietary approach to stop hypertension'. It is a diet which keeps a heart healthy and has been formulated for people suffering from high blood pressure, so that it can keep the blood pressure under control. This diet comprises all types of grains, fruits, vegetables, dry fruits and low-fat/fat-free dairy products. During the course of this diet, a check is imposed on such foods and beverages which contain sweet, red meat and fat. This diet enhances the quantity of potassium, calcium, magnesium and other nutrients in your body. These elements help in lowering blood pressure. The study has revealed that blood pressure starts to nosedive within two weeks of initiation of this diet and within two months, cholesterol level in the blood comes down. During the DSH diet, intake of salt should be limited in order to make this process more effective. Avoid junk foods.

Genie Craig Diet

Genie Craig diet plan is the one that controls calories and fat. In this diet, more emphasis is laid on fruits, vegetables, all types of grains, low-fat dairy products and healthy fat foods. This diet also comprises of lean meat, poultry, fish, *dalia,* eggs and dry fruits. In this diet plan, there is prohibition of junk food and soda. It is a balanced diet plan which can be implemented easily and you need not count your calories during this period.

Learn Diet

In this type of diet, 60 percent of energy is supplied by carbohydrates and less than 10 percent of energy is obtained from fats. 'Learn Diet' means Lifestyle, Exercise, Attitude, Relationship and Nutrition. This diet plan comprises of fruits, vegetables and beans. As far as possible, keep away from fatty foods. This diet supplies good amount of good carbohydrates. In addition, rich-fat foods are strictly prohibited.

Weight Watchers' Diet

Under weight watchers' diet, the members help people

control their eating habits and practices as well as stress more of physical exercise. Under this diet plan, fat foods are strictly prohibited. More stress is laid on steamed vegetables, fruits, salad etc. Weight watchers adopt a modern approach.

Slim Fast Diet Plan

This diet plan works on 3-2-1 formula. It comprises of fruits and vegetables, while junk foods and calorie-rich foods are prohibited. This diet plan can be adopted at any place and time.

Ornish Diet

This is a vegetarian diet plan based on low fat, which encourages lower weight with cultivation of capability to fight heart ailments and cancer. Meditation, exercise and group support are recommended under this program. Food can be taken up at any time, which comprises fruits, vegetables, beans and grains. It also includes rich-fat foods and low-fat dairy products. There is strict prohibition on the things which do not suit your body, such as wine, red meat, cold drinks, fat, oil, sugar and salt. As you eat frequently at short intervals, you get enough energy and the metabolic rate improves too, which in turn helps to burn calories and lose weight.

□

33
How to Eat

- Never begin the day with coffee or tea. The food articles with caffeine only increase blood pressure and heart rate. It makes you feel stressed, which is the greatest enemy of the digestive system. When we drink tea or coffee in the morning, it feels like we are fresh but actually heart beat and breathing rate had increased. The body is quite light in the morning hours, and the heart beats at a normal pace. To maintain this normal pace, what we need is the real food. Tea or coffee gives only negligible amount of nutrition to the cells hungry for the last 9-10 hours. Drinking tea or coffee only kills appetite and you can stay hungry for over a long period of time without actually feeling it. With sunrise, metabolism is at its peak. It is the time when you need to eat something. If you don't want to eat solid at this hour, you can have fruits. One hour after this, you can eat fibrous food, like chapatti, upama, idli, poha etc. Once, cells have been supplied with nutrition, you can follow it up with tea or coffee.
- Eat after every two hours. It will not allow you to go obese, rather it will reduce your amount of eating. When you consume fewer calories at one time, they will be utilized in a better way and will not get collected in the body. Eating at short intervals makes the body feel better.
- Eat as per your activity; if you are more active, eat more; if you are less active, eat less. If keeping hungry is a punishment, eating more is surely a crime. We keep eating

without paying attention to the needs of our stomach and body. We get bulky because we prefer to eat at wrong times. For example, a sweet like laddoo has a lot of calories, and if it is eaten along with food or at night, then you cannot prevent it from being stored in the body as fat. After you have eaten to the full and after the rate of metabolism has slowed down (after sunset), the body rejects nutrients. A sound and stress-free sleep too helps to melt away fat. The right way is to eat your full meal by half past six and a light meal at half past eight at night. Your body requires more of calories during stress, illness and travel.

- You can consume poha, dhokla, salad, sprouted dals, fruits etc., but avoid oil and sugar. The consumption of carbohydrates only stimulates your appetite, so include proteins also in your diet.
- Eat seasonal fruits and vegetables. It is better to eat whole fruits in place of fruit juices. Different vegetables supply different types of nutrients. Eat green leafy vegetables a lot as they have enough minerals and vitamins.
- If you wish to lose weight, reduce intake of white items, such as potato, maida, sugar, rice, etc., and lay emphasis on multi-grains and multi-fruits, such as dals, wheat, gram, barley, carrot, spinach, apple, papaya, etc.
- Consume fat-free milk and curd. It is better to remove cream (malai) in place of mixing water in the milk. Mixing water only reduces the amount of nutrients in it. You can eat paneer and curd made from soya. Those who are susceptible to the allergy of milk or soya products should consume rajma, lemon, tomato, methi (fenugreek), almond, cashew nut in order to avoid deficiency of calcium.
- Have 3-4 litres of water or other beverages every day. Water not only helps to lose fat, but remove toxins from the body also. It reduces appetite and prevents constipation. Start eating meals with a glass of water, coconut water, juice, soup, lemon water or buttermilk.

□

34

Shrinking Age, Expanding Waist

Often people find themselves busy trying to lose weight but do you know that it is more important to shrink the waist and stomach than to lose weight? You can certainly lose weight somewhat easily but the most terrible problem is to lose fat from around the waist and stomach. You might know a few people who are not otherwise obese, but they have a lot of fat round their stomach, which is a source of trouble for them and they think themselves as obese. This has adverse impact on girls and women who cannot put on tight clothes for the fact of accumulated fat around waist and stomach regions. If they do, they don't look pretty enough and their

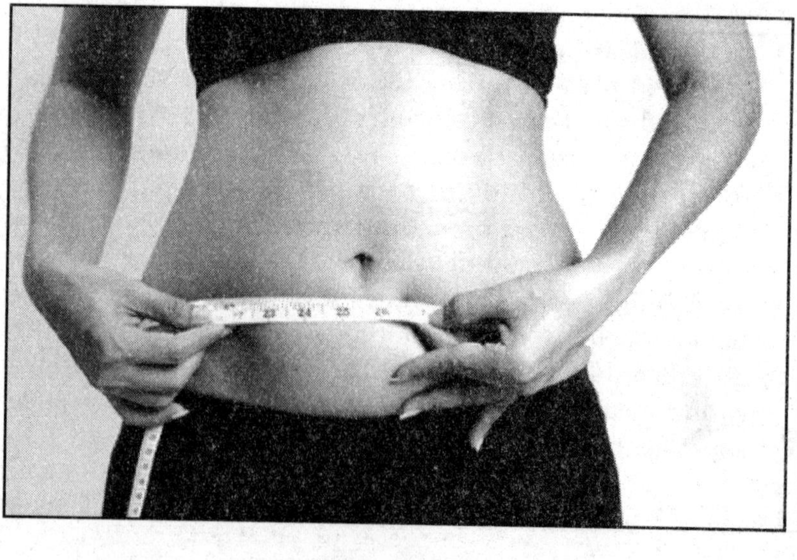

personality does not seem to be impressive. If you wish your waist and stomach to shrink easily, then a few of tips can be very handy for you.

Come, let us discuss few tips for shrinking waist and stomach size:

Fast once a Week

If you are fond of eating and you are perturbed by this habit of yours, its better you observe fast once a week. If you desire, you can stay on liquid diet once in a week. During this, you should prefer water, lemon water, milk, juice, soup etc. If you wish, you can limit your diet with salad or fruit only on one day. Eating salad will certainly help you lose weight.

Yoga is Essential

To bring waist and stomach under control, you should practise yoga daily in the morning. You should include such asanas in it which help to shrink these body parts of yours. Moreover, yoga helps you stay healthy and free from diseases. All actions of the Surya namaskar are very effective, besides you can do sarvangasana, bhujangasana, vajrasana, shalabhasana, etc.

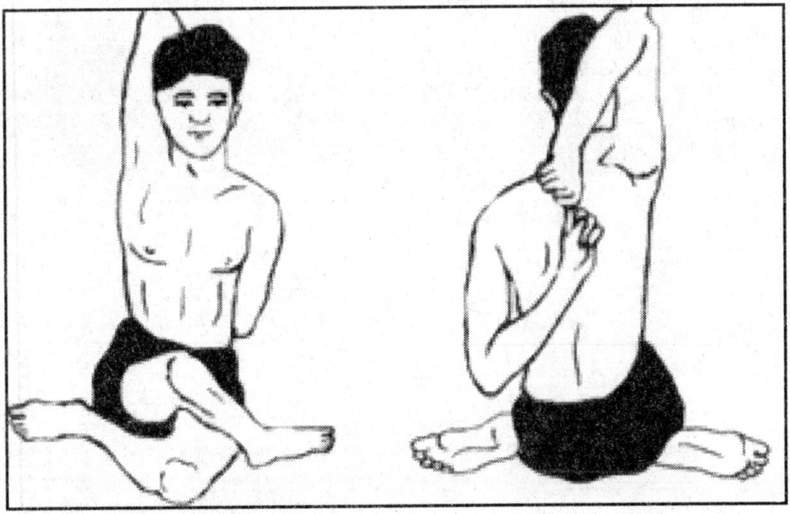

Control Eating

If you are fond of eating junk or oily food, then you must control this liking. Prefer chapatti prepared from mixed barley-gram flour, rather than ordinary wheat flour. It will help tone up your body.

Honey is Good

Honey possesses a lot of good qualities and is helpful in shrinking the waist size. You should consume honey with water daily morning. It will help you reduce the waist and stomach size.

Green Tea is Helpful

If you are fond of drinking tea a lot and still wish to lose weight, then you should replace your milky tea with green tea, lemon tea or black tea. These are full of antioxidants. In fact, milk in the tea increases the possibility of weight gain.

Walk in Morning and Evening

To remove fat from your waist and abdomen, you should go for a walk in the morning; and never forget to go for a stroll after dinner. It will help you burn extra calories and the fat round your waist and abdomen will get a beating.

□

35

How to Select a Gym

Fitness has become necessary as well as more of a fad in the modern times. Many methods are available for this purpose right from yoga, aerobics to dance therapy. One of the popular methods is gym (gymnasium); however, you must keep in mind that you should select one which follows the right practices and procedures.

The pertinent question is what all things and facilities should be available in a gym. It is clear that a gym should be equipped with different types of facilities and equipments. It should also have trained and skilled trainers, cafeteria for beverages, dieticians and personal trainers etc. It's equipment

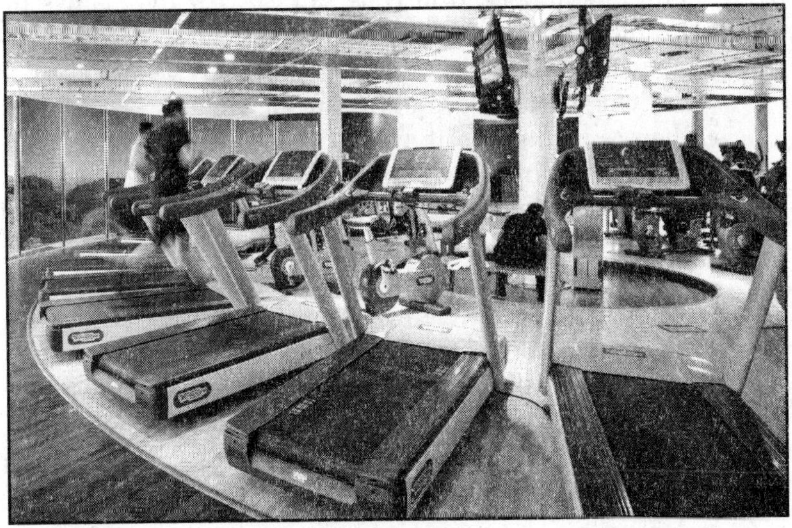

should be branded. If you think all these things make up an ideal gym, then you are possibly wrong. In fact, all these things are essential, but no gym can become an ideal gym with only these.

Before joining a gym, pay attention to a number of points, including the following:

- While selecting a gym for yourself, keep in mind that it should be as per your lifestyle; should support your lifestyle. It should not merely contribute or play the role of a medical treatment.
- A gym may be joined by the youth as well as people of middle age. The youth join a gym especially for body building, while some people become its member to stay fit. Everybody has a unique body constitution. Level of health condition varies too. Few are heart patients and few suffer from high blood pressure. A gym should be equipped with different types of programmes as per each member's requirement. Therefore, it is essential that a gym has the services of a professionally trained trainer/coach.
- The equipment being used in a gym should be branded as well as of good quality. Such equipment will help undertake physical exercises in a proper manner. Equipment should also be safe so that they cause no harm to muscles and body; further they prevent the occurrence of any accidents.
- A gym should focus on balancing the body fat, rather than reducing obesity.
- Those who join a gym for the first time should adopt an exercise regime and nutrition regime which is short in the beginning and that can be completed as per physical capability.
- You can be inclined towards physical work only when there is an adequate and suitable environment around. Cleanliness, hygiene, positive attitude of workers and people keep your interest alive as well as fresh.
- While selecting a gym, keep in mind that you need its services to keep both body and mind fit. There should

be facilities of massage, steam, shower, health juice café etc. so that you can de-stress yourself there itself.

- A gym should have a professional consultant, fitness specialist, dietician etc. in order to guide you properly as it may be pertinent to your health condition and need. A specialist should guide according to the body needs, health problems and dietary needs.

□

36

Regular Exercise

Obesity gives you a shapeless body as well as a home for illnesses and ailments. Of course, obesity brings with it a number of ailments. The root cause of diseases like diabetes, heart condition, high blood pressure, excess of cholesterol and the like is nothing but obesity. When you are obese, you tire out sooner than later; you breathe heavily and have to stop working. The most suitable method to reduce obesity is to undertake a regular exercise regimen. Exercise not only reduces your weight but keeps you agile and active also. It makes you feel good.

Walking

Walking is the most effective and simplest exercise which doesn't require you to plan your time separately. You can make walking a part of your daily routine quite easily.

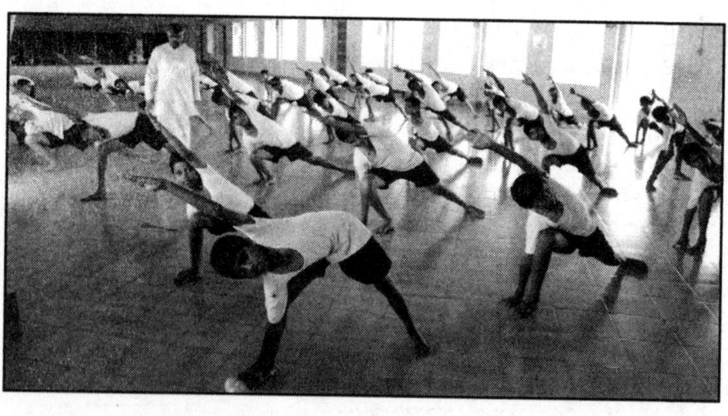

Use Stairs

If you shy away from taking to stairs and prefer the lift, better change your attitude. The most essential way to reduce obesity is to do physical work, so use more of stairs than the lift.

Walk to Nearby Places

Avoid driving or riding a vehicle if you are headed for a nearby place, until it is not absolutely necessary. Try to walk. Walking for an hour a day melts away your extra fat.

Cycling

Cycling is a good physical exercise to reduce fat. It can help you remove your extra fat collected in your body. Cycling for half an hour a day in the morning will make you feel the change.

Swimming

You can swim to lose weight. Swimming uses up a lot of calories, so this is an adequate exercise for weight loss. A few days after you start swimming, you will see for sure that your weight is descending down the scale.

Skipping

Skipping a rope is a good exercise. It helps you to burn your fat rapidly. Besides, it gives you stronger leg muscles.

Jogging

Rise early in the morning for jogging. It will help you to reduce weight as well as keep the body agile and fit. Jogging for an hour daily is quite helpful in losing weight and controlling obesity.

□

37

Manage Carbohydrates

Eating junk foods and fast foods aggravates the problem of obesity. The carbohydrates found in these foods contribute significantly in gaining obesity. If you eat more of carbohydrate-rich food, such as chapatti, cake, potato etc., the threat of obesity multiplies. You can keep your weight under control by avoiding carbohydrate-rich foods; however, if you make carbohydrates disappear from your diet altogether, then it has a negative impact on the brain. Vegetables, fruits, soup, juice and cucumber salad should be eaten regularly. Doing this will not allow you to gain weight, nor will it expand your stomach-line and will give you enough energy.

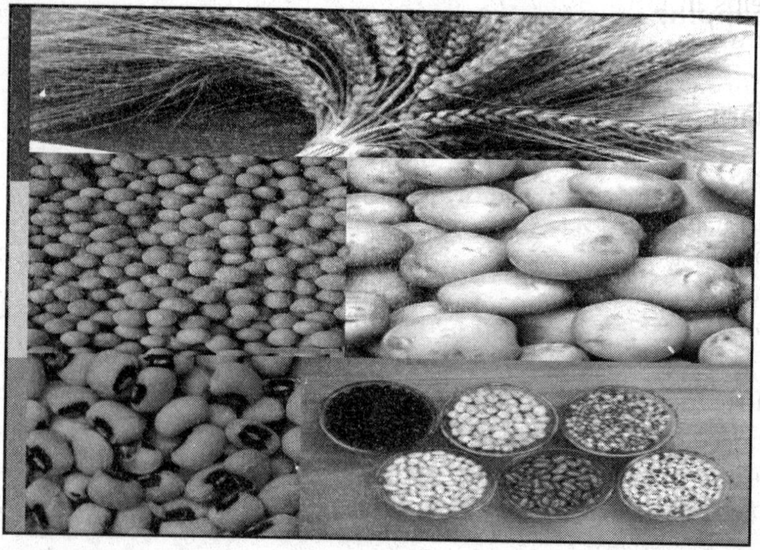

What Is Carbohydrate?

Carbohydrate is a carbonic product which comprises carbon, hydrogen and oxygen. The ratio of hydrogen and oxygen is like the ratio of water. Carbohydrate works to provide heat and fat to the body. The body gets the supply of carbohydrates in two ways – in the form of starch and in the form of sugar. Starch is found in wheat, barley, corn, bajra, raw grains, rice, pulses and root vegetables.

More carbohydrate is found in banana, guava, sugarcane, chukandar (beetroot), khajur (date), munakka (currant), anjeer (fig), sugar, honey, sweet vegetables and almost all sweet foods which are all very powerful and good for health. Their excess in the body can cause many harmful diseases, like diarrhoea, diabetes etc. Carbohydrate-rich foods cause to gain weight at a tremendous rate.

Benefits of Consuming Carbohydrate

Consuming 20 gm of carbohydrates everyday in food maintains the body energy because these are main sources of energy in the body. It also supplies the brain with sufficient quantity of glucose and this helps the brain function better and effectively. Consumption of carbohydrate-rich food also helps in normalising blood sugar level, which helps to bring down appetite.

Harm of not Consuming Carbohydrates

Carbohydrate-rich diet results in weight gain and in view of this, there are people who reduce or stop its consumption. Such people are affected mentally because avoidance of carbohydrate-rich food cuts off supply of glucose to the brain. In such a situation, the brain is unable to think and memorise things.

How to Limit Carbohydrate in Diet

We can control our obesity by limiting the quantity of carbohydrates in our daily diet. Avoid those things which are abundant in carbohydrates but it is not at all advisable to stop such things all of a sudden or completely. Sometimes, people are prone to think that carbohydrates do nothing but increase fat while they forget that it provides our body with essential energy. For this, you can shift to the alternatives of bread, chapatti etc. Therefore, you can adopt such foods which have less of carbohydrates, such as vegetables, fruits, soup, juice and salad.

□

38

Do Garudasana to Lose Weight

Practising yoga makes it possible for all ailments to be treated and if you are suffering with obesity, yoga can prove to be the easiest method to lose weight. Yoga can be done quite easily. There are a number of yogaasans to lose

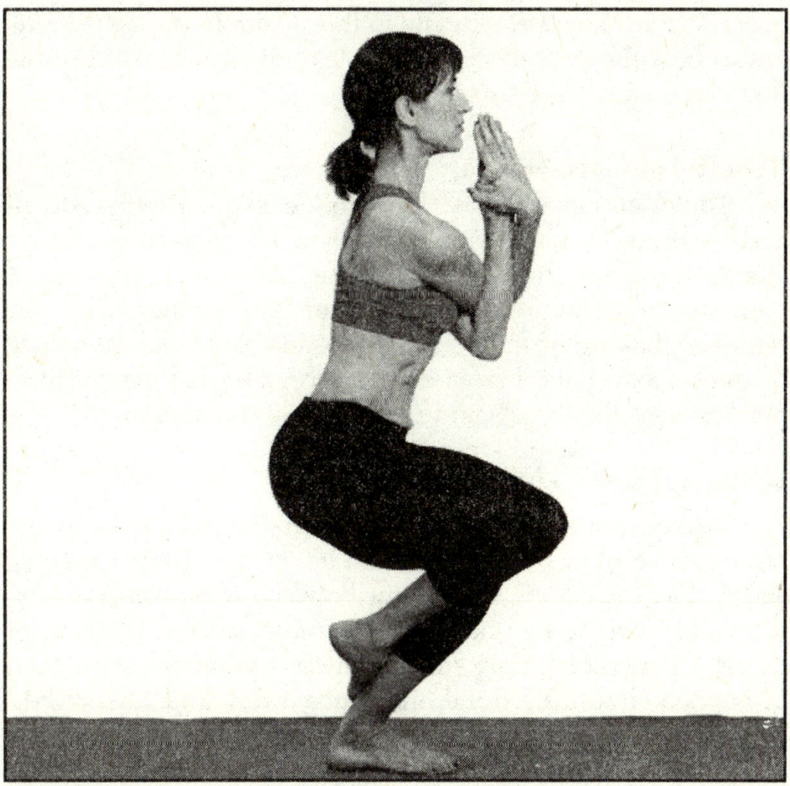

weight, such as trikonasana, konasana, uttanapadasana, pavanmuktasana, Surya namaskar, Garudasana and so on. Of these, Garudasana is a very simple posture. It is good to reduce obesity. This asana is beneficial to the people who suffer from kidney disorders or feel pain in hands and feet. If there is any deformity in legs, this aasan can be of great help.

Garudasana

In this asana, an individual takes the shape of a Garuda, a large eagle-like bird (mount of Lord Vishnu in Hindu mythology). It is essential to focus the mind in this aasan. First stand straight in attention and then taking the right leg from the front, wrap it round the left leg. In the same manner, wrap both the hands before the chest and fold them in the position of Namaskar. Hold it for a few moments taking breath and then come to normal position. After a breath, repeat the same process from the other side. Be in this position for one minute, and repeat the process with both legs five times. With time, you can increase the duration.

Benefits of Garudasana

This asana helps to make the spine flexible, waist slims down and the muscles and veins of arms and legs become active. Hands, knees and thighs become strong. This yoga also rectifies pain and trembling of shoulders, arms and elbows. This also removes shaking of the body. This asana also helps to reduce backache, joint pain, hernia etc. This yoga is very beneficial in obesity, piles, hydrocele and urine-related diseases.

When to Do

While undertaking Garudasana, make sure to keep the body clean and fresh. There should not be any kind of fatigue. This yoga can be done at any time between sunrise and sunset. It should be done two hours before meals or four hours after meals. Doing it on empty stomach helps to slim down quickly. This yoga should be done only once a day and this should continue for at least 15 minutes but should not exceed one hour at a stretch. If you think to do it over one hour, then divide the period into two sets of 30 minutes, with a brief interval in between. This brief interval should be of 30 minutes.

Avoid Eating

The most important factor to reduce obesity is to change your eating habits. Without taking care of eating habits and type of food, you cannot lose weight. During the period of yoga, you should eat light, easily digestible food and it should not be much fried. Avoid spices and condiments in cooking. If possible eat nutritious food that include green vegetables, salad, milk, butter, etc. This type of food is good for the body. Always stop short of your appetite. Food should be chewed well and for long. Stop taking any tea and coffee during the course of Garudasana.

□

39

Drink Protein Shake to Lose Weight

There are a number of misconceptions and myths when it comes to losing weight. Some people think that they can easily lose weight if they don't eat food. But this is merely a myth. This is quite true that not eating food will lead to loss of weight but this remains effective only for a short period. You might know that the people who starve themselves to lose weight, they gain still more weight later. In fact, you can adopt the formula of starving over a long period of time. When you resume your normal eating after the period of starvation, you will suffer more harm than good. Then the moot point is – What should be done to lose

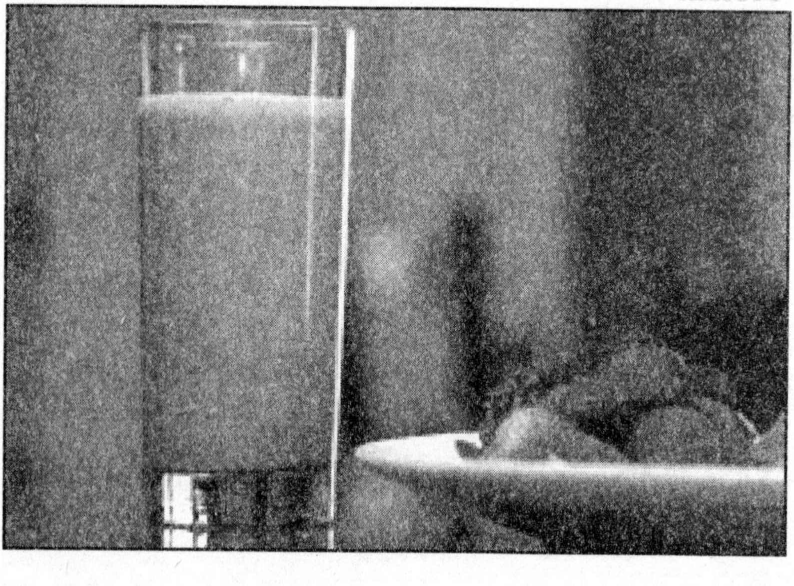

weight? Come, let us find out how we can lose weight by using protein shake.

What Researches Suggest

- In the fast-paced life of modern times, everybody wishes to keep fit but you should remember that it is more important to take a balanced diet rather than starving.
- The recent research infers that you cannot lose weight merely by controlling diet.
- The research also reveals that eating less has no relevance with losing weight.
- The research tells that what you eat determines whether you will lose or gain weight.
- If you reduce the number of calories in your food, your weight will not go down. If you wish to lose weight in a healthy manner, then you should take protein shake.
- According to another research, the women who take protein shake look more beautiful and fresh and are in a position to lose weight within a year when compared with other ordinary women.

Protein Shake to Lose Weight

- Proteins should be taken in sufficient quantity to lose weight and stay fit. It gives you health, as well as strengthens your muscles.
- Protein shake works as a supplement to lose weight. This should be taken in different quantities.
- Take a glass of milk daily, to take protein shake.
- If you wish to lose weight hurriedly, you can also consume protein powder.
- Soya milk is a better protein shake. If you take it regularly, you will find your weight entering within the control limits.
- If you wish, you can also take protein juice.
- If you want to take domestic protein shake, you can mix skimmed milk powder, milk and eggs.

□

40

Adopt GM Diet to Lose Weight

You can try GM diet programme to lose weight and keep fit. The GM or General Motors diet programme has been specifically prepared for the purposes of weight loss. In this program, the menu for all foods to be eaten on different days of a week has been given. If you follow this seven-day diet program, you can find the difference within two months.

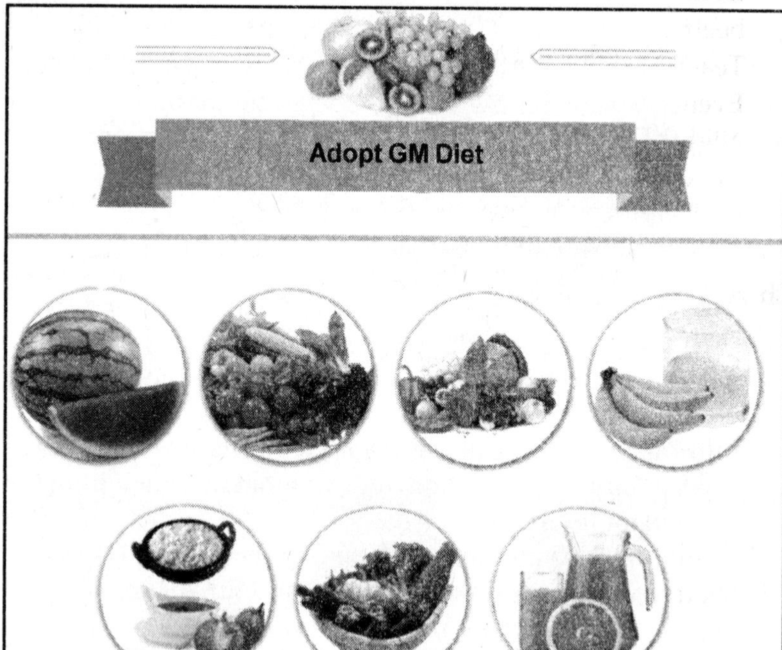

First Day

Breakfast (8.30-9 am): 1 apple, 2 glasses of water.

Mid-morning meal (10.30-11 am): 1 bowl papaya, 2 glasses of water.

Lunch (1-1.30 pm): 1 bowl water melon, 2 glasses of water.

Tea-Time (4-4.30 pm): Orange, lemon or cheeku, 1½ glasses of water.

Evening (6-6.30 pm): 1 glass of coconut water.

Night (8.30-9 pm): 1 apple, 2 glasses of water.

Remember to eat only fruits on the first day but avoid banana.

Second Day

Breakfast (8.30-9 am): 1 boiled potato, 1-2 glasses of water.

Mid-morning meal (10.30-11 am): 1 bowl cabbage, 2 glasses of water.

Lunch (1-1.30 pm): 1 tomato, 1 cucumber, half boiled beetroot, 1½ glasses of water.

Tea-Time (4-4.30 pm): 2 tomatoes, 1-2 glasses of water.

Evening (6-6.30): 1 glass spinach-tomato juice.

Night (8.30-9 pm): boiled lauki (bottle gourd) mixed with salt or spice, 2 glasses of water.

Remember to eat only vegetables on the second day.

Third Day

Breakfast (8.30-9 am): 1 apple, 2 glasses of water.

Mid-morning meal (10.30-11 am): 1 bowl papaya, 2 glasses of water.

Lunch (1-1.30 pm): 1 tomato, 1 cucumber, half boiled beetroot, 2 glasses of water.

Tea-Time (4-4.30 pm): 1 orange, 2 glasses of water.

Evening (6-6.30): 1 glass spinach-tomato juice or 1 cheeku.

Night (8.30-9 pm): boiled lauki mixed with salt or spice, 2 glasses of water.

Remember to eat only fruits or vegetables on the third day.

Fourth Day

Breakfast (8.30-9 am): ½ glass skimmed milk, 2 glasses of water.
Mid-morning meal (10.30-11 am): 1 banana, 2 glasses of water.
Lunch (1-1.30 pm): 1 glass skimmed milk without sugar, 2 glasses of water.
Tea-Time (4-4.30 pm): 1 banana, 2 glass water.
Evening (6-6.30): 1 banana.
Night (8.30-9 pm): ½ glass skimmed milk without sugar.
Remember to take only skimmed milk and banana on the fourth day.

Fifth Day

Breakfast (8.30-9 am): 1 bowl brown rice, 2 glasses of water.
Mid-morning meal (10.30-11 am): 2 tomatoes, 2 glasses of water.
Lunch (1-1.30 pm): 1 bowl brown rice with tomato gravy, 2 glasses of water.
Tea-Time (4-4.30 pm): 2 tomatoes with salt-zeera, 2 glasses of water.
Evening (6-6.30): 1 glass of lemon water.
Night (8.30-9 pm): 1 bowl brown rice.
Remember to take only brown rice and tomato on the fifth day.

Sixth Day

Breakfast (8.30-9 am): 1 bowl brown rice, 1-2 glasses of water.
Mid-morning meal (10.30-11 am): 2 tomatoes, 2 glasses of water.
Lunch (1-1.30 pm): 1 bowl brown rice with other vegetables, 2 glasses of water.
Tea Time (4-4.30 pm): 2 cucumbers with salt-zeera, 2 glasses of water.
Evening (6-6.30): a glass of lemon water.

Night (8.30-9 pm): boiled beetroot, cucumber, carrot, tomato, cabbage salad.

Remember to eat only brown rice and tomato with vegetables on the sixth day.

Seventh Day

Breakfast (8.30-9 am): 1 bowl brown rice, 2 glasses of water.

Mid-morning meal (10.30-11 am): 2 tomatoes, 2 glasses of water.

Lunch (1-1.30 pm): 1 bowl brown rice with other vegetables, 2 glasses of water.

Tea-Time (4-4.30 pm): 2 cucumbers with jeera-salt, 2 glasses of water.

Evening (6-6.30): 1 glass shikanji or any other juice.

Night (8.30-9 pm): boiled beetroot, cucumber, carrot, tomato, cabbage salad.

□

41
Dietary Myths

Calories Have No Importance

This is a misconception. This myth is commonly used in the business pertaining to weight loss. The fact remains that calories occupy a very vital place in losing or gaining weight. To lose 1 pound of body fat, you have to reduce 3,500 calories from your diet. However, when you eat a diet containing fats and common proteins and carbohydrates, you need not count your calories.

Weight can be Lost by Fresh Diet

This is a false myth. To lose weight, it is essential to undertake regular exercise and physical work. Exercise helps to consume and burn calories already present in the body and it helps to control the appetite control system in the brain. Exercise also helps to improve metabolism, control blood pressure and improve health.

Eating More in the Morning than Evening Helps to Lose Weight

This is a false myth. The body does not distinguish between morning or evening hours when it comes to digest food. Your weight is determined by the number of calories consumed.

Calories are Burnt by Eating Things like Grapes

This is a false impression. During the digestion process,

the body gets energy from the foods eaten but there is no food the energy from which can help to control weight.

Don't Stop Smoking to Prevent Obesity

This is a false conception. The weight gained during the initial period after quitting smoking can be reduced using balanced diet and exercise. However, the harm done to lungs and heart by smoking can never be made up.

Slow or Fast Eating Have no Impact on Weight

This is a wrong notion. When a person eats every morsel chewing it well, the body's metabolism can regularise the system in the brain that controls appetite and it can help to reduce hunger. The appetite system in the brain can be satisfied by eating slowly and enjoying food well. This helps to get satisfaction even with less amount of food. Eating fast does not increase weight. Obese people eat in a hurry so they don't give a chance to appetite control system to control things. This further enhances their desire to eat more.

□

42

How the Elderly Can Lose Weight

The Elderly Gain Weight Easily

- With the advancement of age, weight also gets a boost because the process of metabolism gets a beating.
- An older person needs more time to digest food as compared to a young man.
- As we advance in age, the quantity of certain enzymes is reduced which help in digestion. In such a situation, it becomes difficult to digest fatty foods.
- Fat-rich food can easily increase weight in the old people, because their body cannot digest such food.
- It becomes very difficult for the elderly people to lose weight if they eat fat-rich food.
- A diet having fewer carbohydrates and more fat can be the most harmful for an old person.

Don't Consume More Than 30 gm of Fat a Day

- Each gm of fat contains 9 calories, while there are 4 calories in each gm of carbohydrate and protein.
- Extra fat in the diet can be a breeding ground for diseases like heart ailments, diabetes, cancer, etc.
- When less of fat is included in the diet, the body starts burning the fat already stored in the body and thus, it becomes possible for an old person to lose weight.
- If an old person has to lose weight, he should not consume more than 30 gm of fat a day.

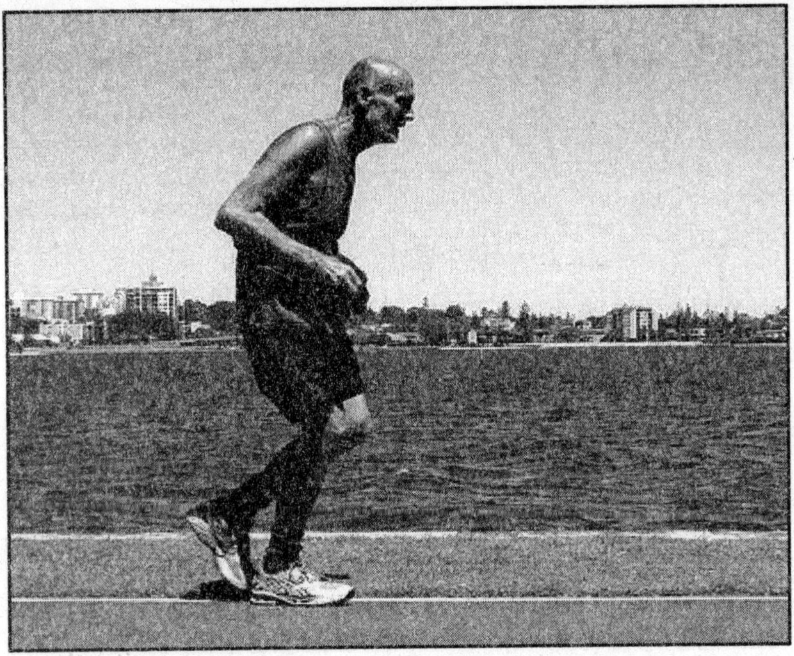

- The table describing the quantity of fat in different foods can be calculated to know how much fat is being consumed a day.

Walk Half an Hour a Day

- To maintain good health and to lose weight without sweating, walking can be an ideal exercise.
- Walking for an hour consumes 3,500 calories. This way, you can lose 1 pound of weight by walking 10 hours.
- Walking helps to improve metabolism process and calories can be burnt rapidly.
- If you walk half an hour a day, enough calories can be spent. If you wish, you can go for a walk 15 minutes at a time both morning and evening.

□

43

Avoid These Mistakes

Everybody is aware that eating more than required and working less than the required exercise by the body pushes us towards obesity. The stomach is like a bank. Whatever we deposit in it gets collected in the form of calories and spend these calories by the work we do. If we deposit more and spend less, more and more of calories will be collected. Thank Heavens, there seems to be no interest being given by this bank.

Come, let us find out the points which can help to control weight.

- Consume fewer calories. If the body gets fewer calories, it would burn the calories already present in it.
- Burn more calories. We can burn them by exercise and work.
- Reduce stress and pressure. People are in want of eating more during stress or pressure. The mistakes we often commit are: eating on fewer occasions but eating more. Often people tend to fill their belly eating once. When we are hungry, we tend to eat stomach-ful without caring for the calories and its result is the increased weight.
- If we take breakfast at 8.30 am and then eat something nutritious at 11.30 am, such as fruits or sprouted grain, then by lunch at 2 pm, we will be less hungry and it will check our eating. In the same manner, don't wait for dinner at night after lunch. You can take two biscuits or roasted gram with tea at 4.30-5 pm. It will mar your

hunger for dinner and you will not be able to eat heavy at night.

- Some people control their diet round the whole week, but at the weekend they eat their stomach-ful then and this leads to their weight gain. They feel that they have eaten limited food all weekdays, and it will not matter much if they eat more on the weekend. But this notion is quite incorrect. If you practise resistance the whole week but consume a great amount of calories at the weekend, all resistance and prevention observed during the week becomes useless.
- Some people love to eat something sweet at the end of their meals but this is not at all right for their health. Carbohydrates are present in the food and eating any sweet after this only harms the body. It increases the quantity of calories abnormally.
- If you are fond of sweets, you can try currant (kishmish), aniseed (saunf) or jaggery (gur). Jaggery supplies iron to the body. Aniseed helps in digestion, while currant does not change into glucose directly.
- There are a number of sugar-free food products in the market. People like to have sugar-free products. It is not advisable to consume sugar-free products in place of natural sweet products over a long time because sugar-free tablets have artificial sweetener which harm the body in the long run. You gain weight when you eat a number of items in small amounts. People tend to think what effect a piece of toffee or chocolate will have on the body but it too provides enough calories to the body. If you are fond of dark chocolate, take only a small piece, or have a wafer chocolate. You can replace *namkeen* (salted fried food) in place of puffed corn, black gram or normal popcorn.

□

44

How to Lose Extra Fat

May be some people have sweated for hours in the gym or have subsided on a cucumber or watermelon in a bid to live. The truth remains that none of sweating to the last bone in the gym or keeping your mouth closed to avoid eating is not the only method to lose weight. In fact, a healthy body needs to cultivate some healthy habits:

Willpower

Your plan to lose weight depends on your determination and attitude. Many people complain that they have not succeeded despite hard exercise and diet control. The fact remains that you can find a way to success only if you are determined to achieve your goal.

Logical Goal

If you plan to reduce 10 kg of weight in three months even when you have never controlled your diet or undertaken physical exercise, it is something beyond reality, nor it is logical and reasonable. In fact, the program, which is not keeping pace with your life style but requires hard work will not help you to lose weight. So, it is better to lose weight gradually. It is not advisable to work in a haste.

Necessary Exercise

Whatever in your age, give enough importance to physical exercise in your daily life. You can adopt any method to exercise, like swimming, playing tennis, walking briskly or aerobics. Nothing can be better if you focus on your waist while doing your household duties. Besides, don't keep doing the same kind of exercises. You can do away with your monotonous exercise regimen by replacing one thing with another. For example, you can replace jogging with swimming or playing tennis. While beginning a new exercise, keep in mind to start with small steps. You can do it for ten minutes in the beginning, and then go on increasing its duration to 30-45 minutes.

Diet Control

To lose weight, you have to control your diet. Eating less can be dangerous. Initially, you can feel some difference, but when you resume your past routine, you will find that you have gained more weight than you actually lost. It is good to enjoy good food and eat sweets but exercise self-control.

Don't be Lazy

If you work hard in the gym but follow sedentary life style then you are sure to gain weight than you lose. The people doing deskwork, face problems when it comes to certain types of exercises. You also have to sit idly while watching television or surfing internet. If you wish to be healthy, walk a lot. If you wish to have a glass of water, fetch it yourself. Use stairs and give up the lift.

□

45

Lose Weight by Surgery

People adopt different techniques to lose weight, so they can look agile and fit; however, some techniques might appear to be costlier. Some people are so upset by their obesity that they decide to go for surgery. The questions arise: Is it safe to undergo surgery to lose weight? Do any techniques adopted to lose weight have evil consequences? Has one to go for repeated surgery to keep weight under control? There are many other questions like these. Let us find out if it is safe to undergo surgery to lose weight.

About the Surgery to Lose Weight

- In fact, surgery is adopted as an option get rid of obesity. The fat is removed from the body part where it has collected greatly. Not only this, the body part where fat is less than required, it can be implanted there too.
- Bariatric surgery is undertaken to remove fat. This surgery is undertaken only on those people who have excess weight by 30-40 kg. An advantage of this surgery is that the body loses 60 kg of weight during six months. In fact, in this surgery, 80 percent part of the stomach is cut off.
- In the present technological age, some people are undertaking such surgeries. Some people undertake surgeries to look slimmer and better.

Advantages of Bariatric Surgery

- Obesity brings a number of other diseases along with it, such as depression, high blood pressure, diabetes. Surgery helps to do away with these.
- The moment obesity is gone, you become more active.
- The problems of peevishness and less efficiency are resolved which are the initial outcomes of obesity.

Disadvantages of Surgery

- While the surgeries undertaken with a purpose to lose weight have certain advantages but at the same time there is a flip side too. You have to improve upon your lifestyle after a surgery for this purpose.
- If you still continue to be lethargic and lazy, you can confront obesity once again.
- This surgery is expensive and cannot be undertaken off the cuff.
- After this surgery, food is hard to digest. Not only this, hunger lessens, as appetite-raising hormone stops working.
- Many people have to undergo this surgery over 2-3 times.

□

46

How to Control Weight in Winters

The winter season means eating time. However cautious you might be regarding your health, the winter season somehow indolence is set in. As a result, there is much possibility of your gaining weight. In such a case, you have to be cautious regarding your daily routine.

Come, let us find out how weight can be kept under control in the winters.

Continue with Exercise Regimen

It is hard to leave bed during winter season. However, you have to emancipate yourself from this trap. It is essential

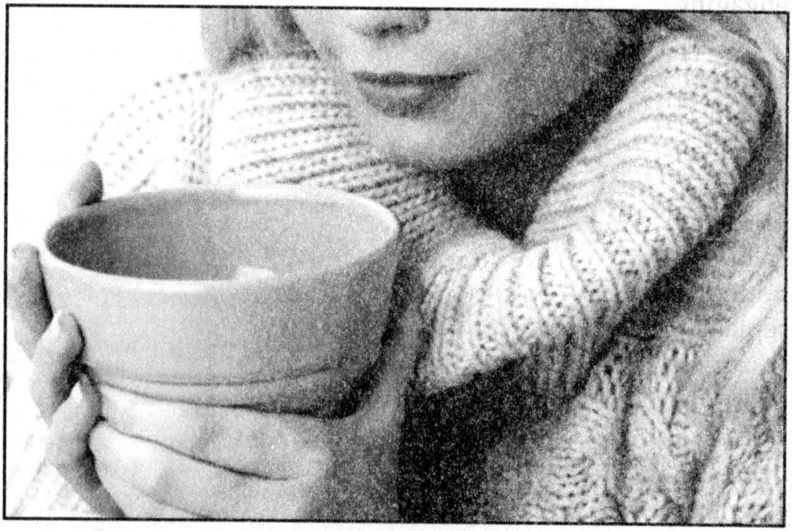

that you don't overlook your exercise regimen during this season. If you are unable to set out of the house for exercise, then take exercise within the four walls of the house, but don't skip it. This is the only method to prevent laziness and weight gain.

Fibrous Diet

You love to eat something or the other when this season is on. You therefore have to be cautious. Whenever you feel like eating, avoid junk food and opt for healthy food. Lay emphasis on fibrous fruits and vegetables. It will make you feel full, while your desire to eat junk food can be kept under control.

Be Active

The desire to work diminishes during this season; however, you can bring about a change in your daily routine in order to keep yourself active. In this way, you can keep your weight under control and remain healthy. For example, if you could not go for a morning walk, don't worry, just go for a stroll in the evening or set out for office a little earlier in order to walk longer. This is the right time to learn some new thing or practise your hobby. You can also keep healthy during winters by engaging yourself in some activities like dance or game.

Control Tea and Coffee

In winters, one is prone to take more of tea and coffee. However fascinating and delicious you might like the cup of hot tea or coffee, yet the presence of nicotine and caffeine are not at all good for your health. These elements boost up calories in the body. As sugar is put in them, tea and coffee is bound to increase your weight quite rapidly. If possible, replace these beverages with lemon or mint tea.

Water is Essential

We seldom feel thirsty in winters, therefore, we hardly drink water in winters. However, keep in mind that water is essential to keep your metabolism active. If you feel that the water cold, you can opt for green tea, herbal tea or black tea. It would be better to leave out sugar from tea.

Wine is Bad for Health

People are in wont of wine in winters, which is not at all good for health. It increases your weight, as well as encompasses you with a number of ailments. If you wish to keep your weight under control, you should not consume much of alcohol; it would save you from gaining extra calories. □

47
Medicines the Culprit

Usually we link weight gain with our eating habits and daily routine but there could be possibly other reasons behind this. One of these could be the medicine that you take in routine. They might be increasing your weight.

1. Steroid

Some life-saving drugs can work to increase your weight. Specialists opine that the steroids drugs given to asthma and arthritis patients can increase weight if taken over a long period of time. Also, the medicines for migraine and epilepsy too cause an increase in weight.

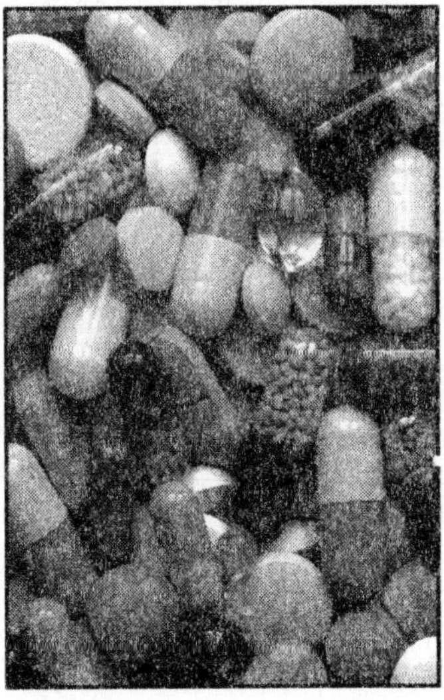

Some people take vitamin or multivitamin tablets, but if these are taken without proper medical advice, there is every danger of not only weight gain, but other illnesses cropping up in the body also. These medicines increase the level of metabolism in the body which has effect on appetite and a person starts to eat more, resulting into an increased weight. However, only these medicines are not responsible for this. Some patients might not take a doctor's advice seriously, and it can lead to the problem of weight gain.

2. Contraceptive Tablets

Sometimes, contraceptive tablets too contribute to weight gain. As a result of these medicines, women often undergo negative impact including weight gain. This weight gain has its effect on a woman's waist, thighs and breasts. Therefore, it is essential that a doctor's advice is sought before starting these tablets.

3. Drugs for Psychological Problems can Lead to Weight Gain

If drugs for depression are taken over a long period, it is possible and vital cause behind weight gain. A psychotic can become aggressive and violent at some time. As a result of such behaviour, it may become essential to administer him with anti-psychotic drugs. These drugs contain chemicals which relax the body and mind, inducing the patient for sleep, and it leads to weight gain. Such patients should keep consulting their doctor so that drugs can be changed as and when necessary. It is also essential for such a patient to undertake regular physical exercise which can help him keep his weight under control.

4. Keep an Eye over Weighing Machine

When you are put on a new medicine or stop taking a medicine, focus on your weight; because abnormal increase or decrease in weight can point to a serious anomaly in the body.

The deficiency of thyroid hormone or hypothyroid too can increase the weight. It is thought that a person normally cannot decrease his weight by more than 10 percent a month, however hard he may work out in the gym or however control he may impose on his diet. For example, if an individual is 70 kg, he cannot lose his weight more than 7 kg in a month. If he starts losing weight more than this, it is a high time to consult a doctor.

□

48

Know Your Metabolism

Our body receives energy from food through a physiological process, called metabolism. This process is a group of different chemical reactions which is created in the organelles of cells in the body. These organelles transform fuel in the food into energy. This energy is utilised in the body in all important processes, such as physical activity, growth, mental reasoning etc. A balanced diet should contain all nutrients necessary for the body, such as carbon, hydrogen, nitrogen, sulphur, phosphorus and other non-carbonic elements. Carbohydrates, fats and proteins supply essential elements to the body.

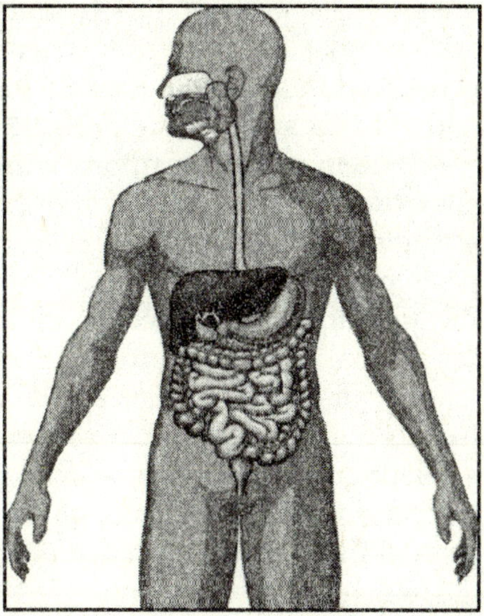

Metabolism is the process of these large particles (carbohydrates, fats and proteins) which are digested, broken into small particles and then oxygenated into small factors. It is only at this stage that these particles are processed by the organelles in the cells and then they get activated by the enzymes and pass through different routes; thus changing into energy.

Carbohydrate metabolism is starch (essence of grain), sucrose (sugar) and lactose (milk sugar). Carbohydrate forms very small parts or units, such as glucose (sugar extracted from grapes), fructose (sugar obtained from fruits) and lactose (milk-related). When food is digested, monosaturides are obtained, which are delivered by the veins from the intestine to the liver. These are then consumed by all the tissues as energy directly. Sometimes they get collected in the liver or muscles in the form of glycogen for some time and can get changed into fat, amino acids or other biological compounds. Generally, carbohydrates provide the body with more than one-half of requirement of energy.

In metabolism of a particle of glucose (sugar extracted from grapes), 31 particles of ATP (main source of energy) are obtained. It is only after this that the energy obtained through ATP is utilized for biological work. The process of carbohydrates metabolism begins with glycosis, obtained from glucose or glycogenesis. The process of changing additional glucose into glycoses is called glycogenesis. This process can take place hours after eating or at night. This process can occur in the liver or muscles in the absence of glucose-6-phosphate.

The process of making glucose from such sources which are not the sources of carbohydrates is called gluconeogenesis. Let us take an example; when carbohydrates are being consumed in a limited quantity in that case certain amount of amino acids and fats are broken down.

Protein contains carbon, hydrogen, oxygen, nitrogen and sometimes other particles too. Metabolism of protein is an essential process. To reach cells, the digestive system breaks protein into amino acids and simple derivative compound. If the quantity of amino acids is more than the quantity required for normal biological process, then they can be used later in 'energy metabolism'. For all the necessary amino acids, the liver is the important place of metabolism. During illness or if a person stays hungry for a long period of time or due to illness; the body does not get enough energy from food, the protein present in the body is broken down.

□

49

Know BMI

This is essential to know what we really mean by being healthy. A simple method to know is BMI or body mass index. The WHO has set the BMI at 25 while the Government of India has set it at 23 because the Indians have 5 percent more fat in their bodies.

How to Calculate BMI

BMI = weight (in kg)/height (in metre)^2

If your weight is 60 kg and height 160 cm or 1.6 metre, then your BMI comes to

= 60/1.6x1.6 = 60/2.56 = 23.4 (that means you are fit).

1. 19 or below: Underweight
2. 23 or less: Healthy
3. 24 to 25: Overweight
4. 26 to 30: Obese
5. 30 or more: Extremely obese

Waist Size Reveals Danger

The BMI is a good method to find out whether you are overweight or not. If your BMI is more than the limit, it simply means that you have more weight than required. However, you might know that if fat gets collected in particular part of the body, it can prove to be more harmful.

The fat collected round the waist is more dangerous than the fat which gets collected in other body parts. If there is more fat round the stomach as compared to other body parts, then there is every possibility of diabetes and heart conditions. To ascertain if there is more than necessary fat round the waist, the waist size is examined, which is as follows:

Women

Normal: 32 inches or less
Excessive: 32–35 inches
Outrageously excessive: 35 inches or more

Men

Normal: less than 37 inches
Excessive: 37–40 inches
Outrageously excessive: 40 inches or more

□

50

How to Lose Weight After Delivery

Women often desire to lose weight and slim down after delivery. This work is not so simple as it might seem. Therefore, women need to adopt a practical attitude if they wish to lose weight after delivery. This requires patience, focus and positive attitude. This objective cannot be realized without bringing positive change in lifestyle.

Diet for Weight Loss after Delivery

- Proper advice and significant exercises contribute to losing weight after delivery. You need to change your diet and eating habits after delivery in order to achieve the objective of losing weight.
- Include fibrous food in your diet. Whole grains, brown rice and fruits are good sources of fibres. Solvent fibre helps to prevent absorption of excessive cholesterol, sugar and starch from the digestive system. Some of

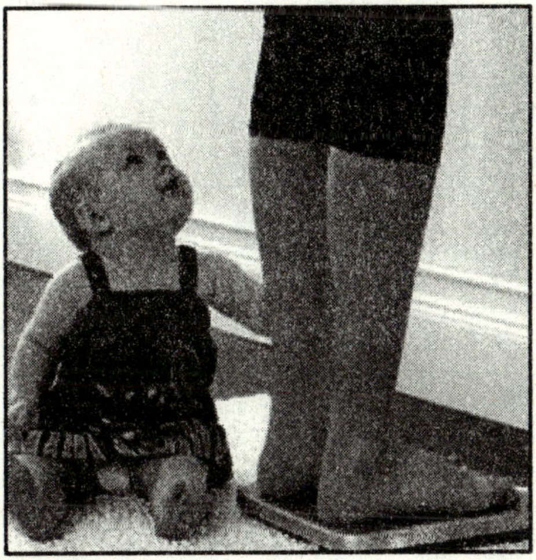

the good solvent fibres are *jai* (millet), *rai* (mustard) and *jau* (barley). Consumption of fibre helps to limit weight after conception.

- Drink lot of water. It helps to extract toxins from the body and it will reduce weight too. Drink water a little before meals. It helps to control appetite.
- Fruits should form an essential part of diet after delivery.
- Have soup thrice a week in order to limit weight gain. This is nutritious as well as helps to reduce calories.
- Avoid chocolate, hot chocolate etc. completely. Chocolate possesses a large amount of calories.
- Make your diet plan. It should include proper quantities of vitamin, calcium, protein, calories, etc.
- Give up junk foods completely.
- If you wish not to work out hard but still wish to lose weight, opt for juice, fruit juice, soup, water and other liquids.
- Eat food two hours before going to bed and always go for a walk after meals. It would help you burn extra calories.
- To limit weight, consume things abundant in antioxidants, rather than taking medicines. Regularly take green tea, lemon tea etc.

□

51

Lose Weight by Yoga

Yoga is the most adequate and simple method to lose weight. The following aasans are useful in losing weight.

Kapalbhati

Throw out air through the nose forcefully. It would make

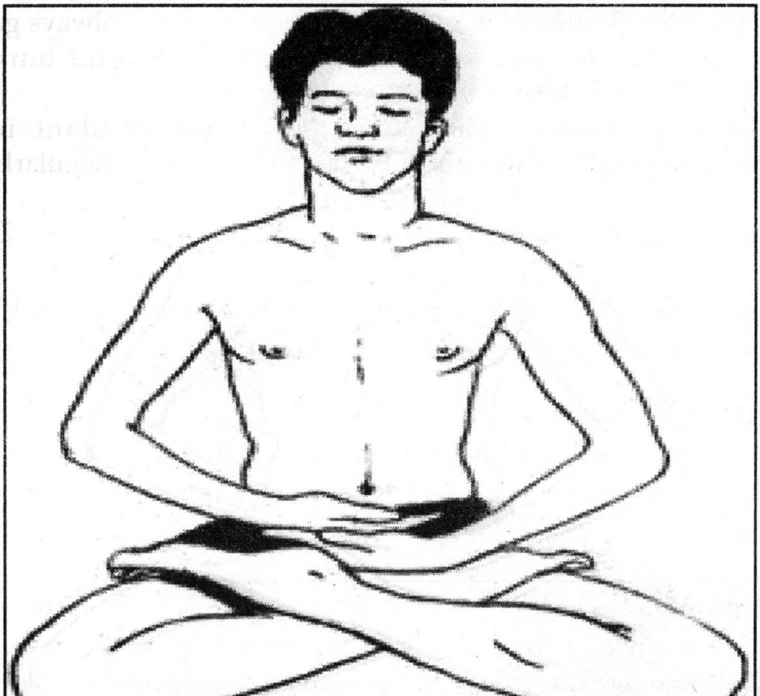

your belly in and out. Do it for 5-10 minutes. Those suffering from high blood pressure should do it but slowly and those suffering from backache should do it on the chair.

Agnisar

Stand with feet opened wide and place your hands on the thighs. Stop out the breath and then pump the stomach, that is, draw in and draw out the stomach. The people suffering from slip disc, high blood pressure or those who have undergone abdominal surgery should avoid this asana.

Urdhva-hastottanasana

Stand with feet apart a little. Lock your fingers of the hand and take them above your head. Breathe out and bow to the left. Repeat the process on both sides.

Drut-uttanapadasana

Lie on your waist and keep your arms under the thighs. Now lift both legs up to 90 degrees. Keep swinging the legs up and down without touching the ground. Those suffering from backache should better avoid it.

Hridaya-stambhasana

Lie on the waist and place hands on the thighs. Breathe in and raise the legs. Also raise your head and waist. During this asana, your body weight will rest on your hips.

Dwipada Cycling

Keep lying on the back. Join your legs and start to rotate them as you do while cycling. Keep doing it until you are tired. Place your hands under the waist.

Bhujangasana

Lie down on your abdomen and place your hands on the hips. Now breathe in and while doing it, raise your head and chest up and turn up towards the back.

Ujjayi Pranayama

This asana is quite beneficial for people suffering from thyroid. Sit straight and breathe out. Now, breathe in and tighten the throat muscles and keep breathing in while making sound from the throat. When full, breathe out through the nose.

□

52
Control Weight after Quitting Smoking

Some people think that smoking too reduces weight and this is the argument that they put forward in order to give some pretense for continuing with it. However, we all are aware how harmful smoking is for our health. How can it be justified to continue smoking just for the sake of our fear of gaining weight?

The most suitable method to control weight is to start physical work and quit smoking. Exercise will keep your weight under control; at the same time, it will keep you safe from terrible health conditions, such as lung cancer, asthma etc.

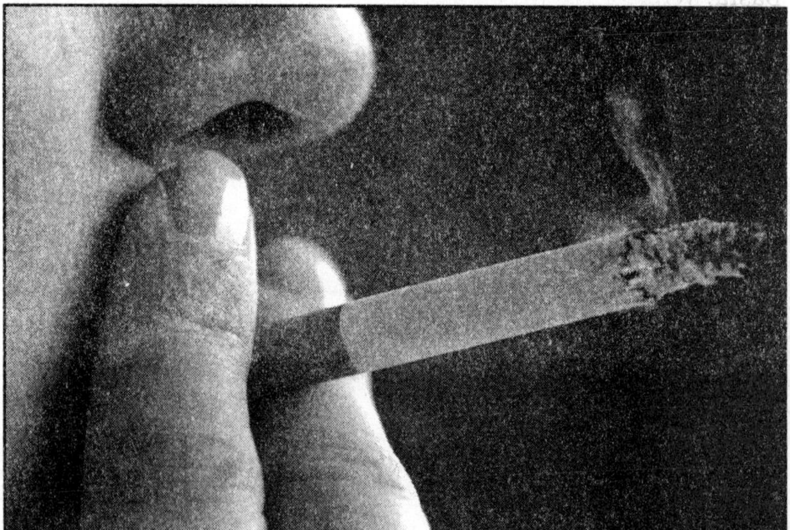

Smoking and Weight Gain

Smoking burns calories in the body. When you quit smoking, your appetite and digestive system become normal, which results in more eating, while the body is unable to burn calories in the same proportion. This results into weight gain too.

When you quit smoking, your capacity to taste food is also increased. After you have quit smoking, you are likely to take snacks in order to quench your appetite rising after quitting the bad habit and it only results in further weight gain.

It is absolutely necessary to undertake physical activity after quitting smoking. Now when you have quit smoking, you need to work a little harder in order to lose fat round your body. If you don't want well shaped muscles then you don't have to sweat hard for this purpose. It would suffice if you walk briskly. The negative side effects of quitting smoking can trouble you for some time and keep you aloof from exercising. Such conditions can be sweating, anxiety, headache, throat swelling etc.

Make a diet plan which contains fruits and vegetables in a sufficient quantity. Eat food in small quantities and avoid meat and other diets which have high amount of calories, like pasta, white bread, white rice etc. Keep away from sugary foods and alcohol too because they contain a large amount of calories.

□

53

Lose Weight by Naturopathy, Ayurveda and Homeopathy

Naturopathy

1. **Massage and Steam:** Sheesham, olive or mustard oil is used for massage. Herbal powder can be used for this purpose. Steam is given after this.
2. **Temperature Bath:** For this, a person is made to sit in water with different temperatures. It helps to relieve constipation.
3. **Special Pack:** Special packs are applied to the body. Mud pack is prepared with mud dug out from two feet below the earth which removes toxins from the body.

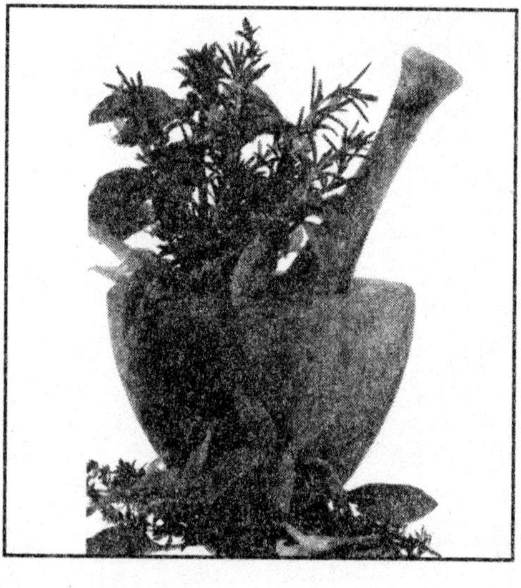

Ayurveda

Ayurveda treatments are chiefly based on herbs and plants. This is much like naturopathy. It also contains techniques like massage and steam bath. For massage, ginger and other herbs are mixed into oil or powder for application and after this, steam is given. Special pack is also used. All these techniques help to melt away fat. In ayurveda practice, up to 5 kg of body weight can be lost in 10-15 sittings. The advantage of ayurveda is that this does not loosen your body, and you do not regain the body weight later. You can also consume trifala, arogyavardhini, ghritkumari and such drugs on medical prescription.

Homeopathy

Have 10-15 drops of Fytolfa Decunda Q or Fucus Vase Q in a quarter cup of water. A person can also take 4-5 tablets of Calferia Carb, thrice a day. These drugs reduce fat, and if taken regularly, they show effect in 2-3 months. These drugs have no side effect. Still, it would bc advisable to consult a doctor.

□

54

Drink Tea Without Milk

People adopt new types of tricks and strategies to lose weight. However, if you attach more importance to the elements that fight obesity, you are sure to lose weight over time. Tea is very beneficial. It keeps you fresh and does away with your indolence. Are you aware that antioxidant present in tea is also effective in losing weight?

- Though antioxidants present in tea help to lose weight,

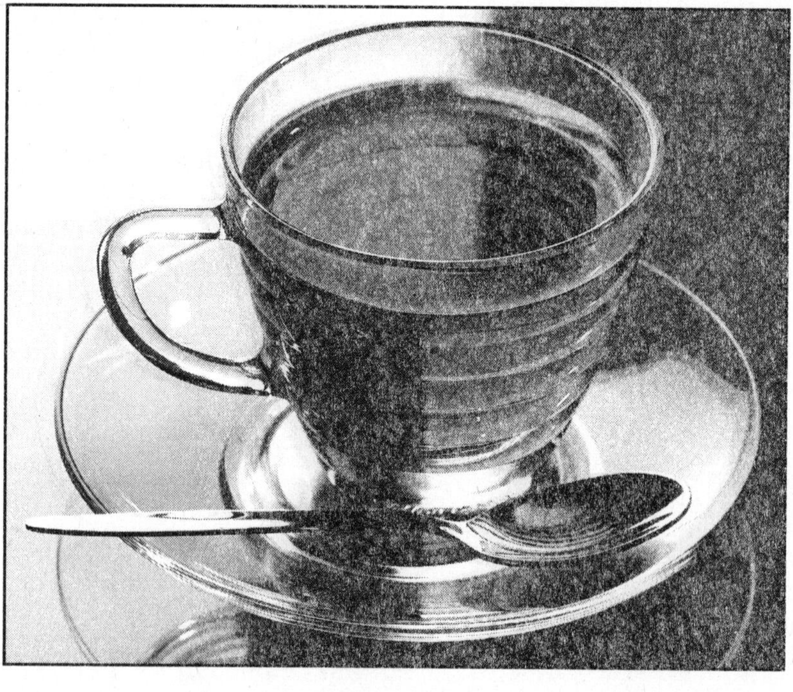

yet milk does away with their benefits. In other words, milk destroys the benefits of antioxidants obtained from tea.

- Milk tea increases weight. Normally, tea contains a number of elements which help to burn fat, but as soon as milk is added to tea, its capacity to reduce weight too goes down.
- There are thepelavins and thirovivins in tea, which are effective in decreasing weight, but milk diminishes their effect. In fact, all these elements are helpful in decreasing body fat as well as decreasing cholesterol. However, milk has more protein in it, which decreases their efficacy.
- Normally tea is beneficial, but when milk is added to tea, the benefits accruing from tea come to an end. The effect of protein present in milk also gets multified.
- If you are fond of tea and wish to lose weight, then never add milk to it. If you go for a practice to the contrary, all your efforts to lose weight will prove futile.
- Milk tea ends all benefits accruing from tea, it also does not benefit your health even an iota.
- Researches have proved that black tea is useful in losing weight and decreasing obesity.

Thus, we can say that milkless tea is beneficial in losing weight. It is also helpful in decreasing the levels of fat and cholesterol.

□

55

Losing Weight by Diet Control is not Good

Those who seek to take help of diet control to lose weight often have negative impact on their health as they have to give up eating and drinking. Dieting never means that you should quit eating altogether and worsen your health. It also makes your skin lose its natural shine; the face seems fatigued and the body listless.

How can a person stay active if he does not eat? The foremost thing to do is to know what ideal weight is for your age and height. For this, consult a doctor and then take further steps. If you can control your weight without dieting, what can be better than this? Weight is also not gained and no need of quitting eating either. For this, you have to adopt some simple methods which can be made part of your daily routine.

- Never include fried items in your food. Avoid them completely.
- Include green vegetables in your diet.
- Manage some time to go for a morning walk.
- Take a glass of lemon water. Potato and rice play a major role in increasing obesity, so limit them.
- Take physical exercise regularly; it will control your weight.
- Timely and sound sleep is very important.
- Avoid cold (aerated) drinks. As they contain a large amount of calories. They are bound to increase your weight.
- Avoid eating sweets in excess.

- Include green leafy vegetables and salad in your diet necessarily.
- Avoid consuming chocolate, pastry, coffee etc.
- Avoid using a vehicle while going to market. As far as possible, walk.
- Try to do your household tasks yourself.

□

56

Domestic Methods to Lose Weight

- After evening meals, set out for a walk with your family.
- Don't sit at a place to watch television. Television is a foe giving obesity. This doesn't burn calories. It only eats away your time.
- Don't watch children playing, join them too.
- Walk not only to the neighbourhood shop, but to the beauty saloon or super market at the next crossing also. Don't look for vehicles for commuting.
- Wash your scooter or car yourself at weekend. Take care of your kitchen garden yourself. Clean your house yourself. If you have nothing else to do, just set photographs in the album. It would be far better than sitting before the television with the remote control in your hand.

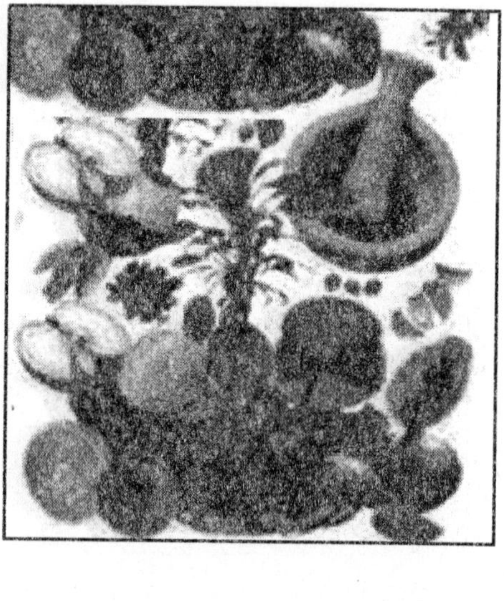

- Sometimes go for an outing with friends to play badminton or other games. Sometimes choose to go for shots in cricket.
- After a bath, go to dry the towel in sun rather than throw it on the

bed. Fold your bed yourself. Instead of asking for water, walk to the kitchen to fetch it yourself.

- Use stairs in place of the elevator.
- If the house has storeys, don't hesitate to walk up and down the stairs.

You might not know that these trivial-looking activities might be greatly helpful in burning extra calories.

□

57
Eat Right to Lose Weight

In the present-day scenario of busy life and stressful lifestyle, everybody seems to be troubled when it comes to the matters pertaining health. The most important factor of this trouble is the carelessness regarding eating habits in daily life. In the fast-paced life of modern times, people have become dependent on fast food, which might feel easier from the viewpoint of cooking and eating, yet such food can only cause a gain in weight as well as harmful effect on the internal functioning.

The most important cause of anxiety for today's youth is their increasing weight. Due to extremely busy daily routine, they are unable to spare time for physical activity or exercise, nor are they able to pay due attention to the nutritional factors in diet. However, if you tend to think that these fast foods and unbalanced diets are the sole cause of increasing weight, you might not know the entire matter. It is also not at all necessary that what you eat at home is always nutritious and balanced and will not cause a gain in weight. Your weight can increase or remain under control and this depends on the fact how you eat food.

If you just swallow your food without chewing every morsel properly, your body weight will increase uncontrollably.

A new research has revealed that if you don't eat chewing well, you will not be able to control your weight despite all kinds of balanced diets and excessive workout in the gym. The researchers have, in this study, found that slim people, as compared with obese people, eat their food chewing well, so they don't gain weight.

An important factor which has been proved right in this research is that women chew their food better than men, while men tend to be careless and in a hurry.

Describing the proper manner of losing weight and eating well, scientists say that if you chew every morsel in your food 35-50 times, it can certainly give you good results. Normally, people chew their morsels not more than 10-15 times.

When you chew every morsel well, you feel yourself mentally and physically healthier. Besides, including raw vegetables and seasonable fruits in the lunch or dinner are good options. When you chew well, the level of your stress goes down. Besides, when you focus on your food, you cannot eat more than you need. It also makes you more satisfied mentally and psychologically.

□

58

Have Good Habits to Lose Weight

If you have tried every trick in the book to control your weight, right from sticking to the strict diet regimen and sweating it out in the gym over long hours and still face failure, there is something wrong with the way you do these things. The specialists are of the opinion that before you adopt all these methods and techniques, you need to adopt good habits. Come, let us find out how you can make your weight control programme successful.

- Success in any undertaking lies in the fact how curious you are about it. It doesn't matter much by saying: "I take so much of exercise but it has no effect." You have to cultivate self-confidence in yourself that you can achieve anything under the sun.
- Never tend to think that you can reduce weight as much as 10 kg in a single month by diet management and physical exercise. Always start at a slow pace and gradually approach your destination. If you adopt kneejerk approach as far as diet management and physical exercise are concerned, you will not be able to regularise it and make it a part of your daily routine. It is, therefore, necessary that for weight control, you should make all those activities a part of your daily routine.

- Take physical exercise regularly. If you feel bored up of one type of exercise, you can take another. Do anything you feel like – tennis, swimming or aerobics. Whenever you initiate a new exercise, begin with a light note of 10-15 minutes and then gradually go on increasing the duration.
- If you undertake physical exercise to keep your weight under control but don't supplement it with active lifestyle, you will not be able to achieve your goal. Therefore, it is advisable to spend more time moving and playing about than watching television or working on computer.
- Crash dieting is not at all good for health. Instead, bring about some positive changes in your diet, such as replacing chips, salted foods and the like with salad and sprouts. Cook your food in little fat. It is better to cook food by baking, steaming than by frying or roasting.

Consume a lot of fibrous foods. Decrease the intake of tea and coffee. Replace these things with lemon water. Take more of vegetables and fruits. Reduce the use of sweet foods. If you are heading for a party, avoid taking fat-rich foods being served there.

□

59

Sleep Well to Lose Weight

Specialists are of the opinion that if you want to lose weight, then you should have sound sleep. The research conducted in the recent times reveals that the people who sleep five hours or less have a heavier frame than those who sleep for seven hours. As per the study those who sleep less; eat more; unable to burn much calories leads to weight gain.

If you want to control your weight, there is no benefit of keeping yourself awake. The earlier researches did not reveal that sleep has any link with weight gain but sleep has always been given a priority. Doctors have been advising sound sleep over ages.

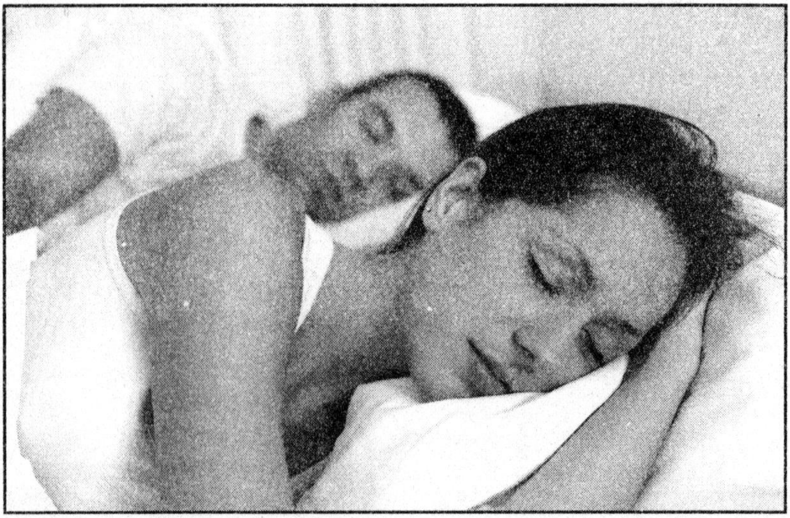

If you sleep enough, the level of your stress goes down; in addition, every organ of the body gets the needed rest. If you keep awake for long hours, the desire to have something or the other will keep creeping up, doing harm to your digestive system as well as body.

As per the research, the people who sleep less eat more calories; besides, their energy is lost due to lack of sufficient sleep which only results into weight gain. On the contrary, those who sleep more, consume fewer calories and burn more energy in sleeping. The study goes on to state that when applied to daily life, sleeping is an important factor of weight gain and obesity.

Insufficient sleep can raise weight, as well as create a number of other problems.

- Insufficient sleep disallows the body to use up carbohydrates completely and it results in an increase of glucose. As a consequence, fat starts getting collected in the body.
- If you sleep less, the level of your lepton goes down, which makes your body desire to eat food rich in carbohydrates.
- Insufficient sleep also decreases the level of hormone excretion which results into a number of problems in the body.
- Insufficient sleep hinders the process of manufacturing of insulin that can result into a higher threat of diabetes.
- Enough sleep can protect you from the threat of high blood pressure.
- Not enough sleep enhances the threat of heart ailments also.

□

60
Plan Diet to Lose Weight

Who doer not want a well-shaped body? It makes our personality attractive and fascinating. On the contrary, obesity is the knock on the door intimating the arrival of a number of diseases. It does not take long to induce obesity but losing weight makes even the most resolute people sweat.

Today, everybody wishes to stay healthy and fit so that he can do all his tasks energetically and swiftly. If we talk of diet control, how can beauty-loving women lag behind? They keep focussing their attention on diet control, all in a bid to have a well-shaped body and infinite charm.

Losing weight is a massive challenge for those whose work is sedentary. If a person works all day sitting on the desk, he is sure to have a heavier weight.

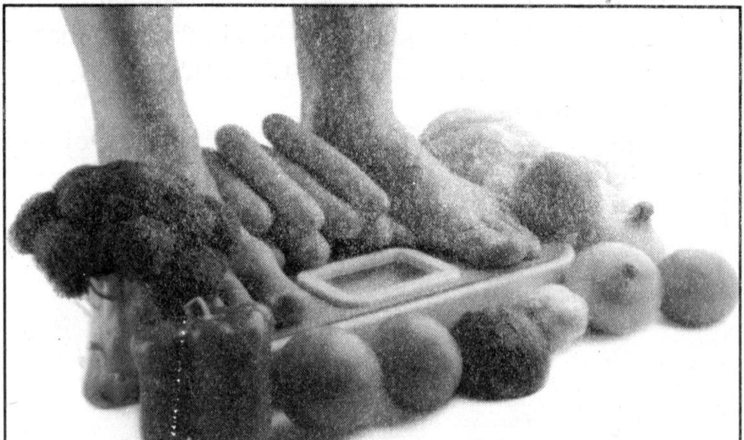

If you are resolute, you can easily lose weight but you will not be able to achieve this if you lack will power and keep postponing your plans and programmes of weight control.

Essential Measures

- Make a diet plan for every day of the week and consume food accordingly.
- Form a habit to have a bowl of soup or salad before eating main course meal.
- If you don't sleep well, you are prone to gain weight as fatigue also causes an increase in weight, so form a habit to sleep and wake up at set times.
- Give up readymade food available in the market, such as pizza, burger or dosa, and adopt home-made food.
- Watching television while eating food is a disastrous habit. It makes you focus your attention on the television and you keep eating even after your stomach is full.
- If you blame party, feasts, weddings and festivals for your weight gain, you are completely wrong. These are part of social life that you cannot avoid but you can certainly avoid eating food that is not good for your health.
- Whenever you feel hungry, go for fruits or vegetable salad. This is beneficial for your health as well as beauty.
- Losing weight never means not to eat, rather it means to have stomach-ful of balanced and nutritious food. Always eat to your appetite.

□

61

Lose Weight Around Waist and Abdomen

For most people, the fat collected round abdomen and waist poses the greatest challenge. It may be the case that you may have a good shapely and slim figure all over the body

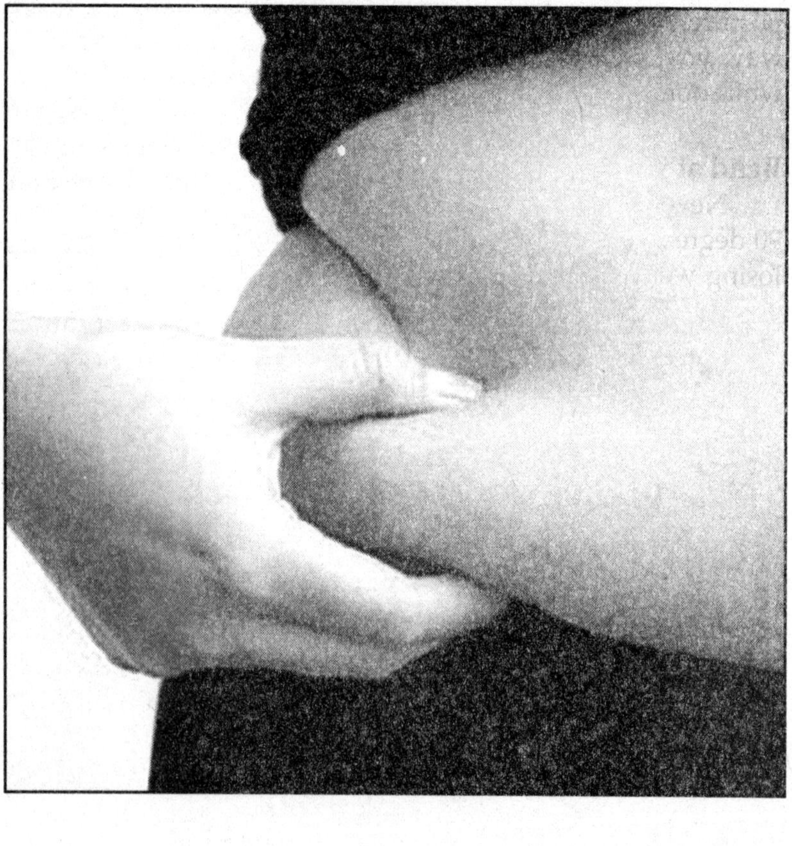

except waist and abdomen. If you are facing this problem, you must adopt four easy measures and then you will see how your obesity evaporates giving you a shapely slim abdomen.

Rotate Shoulders

Rotate your shoulders from forward to backward in turn. It is an ordinary stance of the body and helps to remove fat from round abdomen and waist.

Pull up Your Abs

Pulling abs upwards may be painful but doing this helps to melt away fat quite quickly.

Right Posture

We have always heard our teachers talk about right posture, but normally, we don't follow it in our daily life. Any way, you are not yet late. Pay attention to the right posture while doing different types of tasks. It will help you lose weight.

Bend at 90 Degrees

Never strain your back, rather bow down at an angle of 90 degrees. Don't bend your ankles. This is a good method of losing weight.

□

62
Effective Measures

Some people bind themselves in their daily routine in order to lose weight. Come, we will tell you some small measures to lose weight and decrease obesity, which are quite simple in nature.

Way of Eating

We all might pay attention to what we eat in order to lose weight but the more important factor remains to pay attention to the method of eating food. The right way of eating food is to start with salad and vegetables and then take lunch or dinner.

Consume Protein

Take protein in breakfast. Milk is a good source of protein. So, you can can take a glass of milk in the morning. After having taken protein, you can take snacks, which then do not have so much of adverse impact as it can harm on an empty stomach.

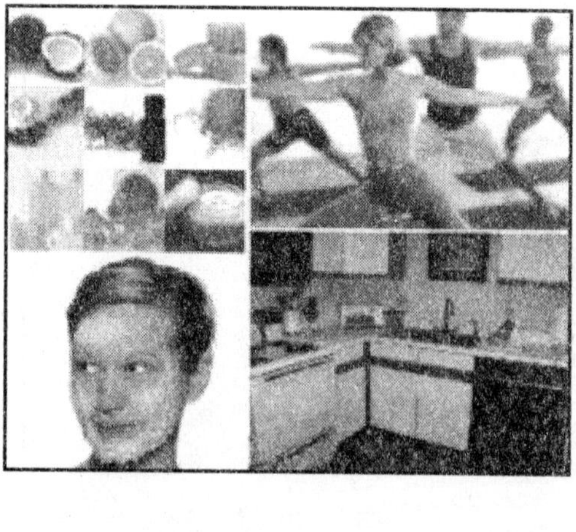

Exercise is also Vital

Make exercise a part of your daily routine and lifestyle.

Do some exercise in the morning as well as evening. It is not at all necessary that you sweat out for hours together. Physical exercise even over half an hour can be sufficient. Do cycling, play games or dance to your favourite tunes.

Fruit Juice

Some people are of the view that fruit juices help in losing weight. If you wish to consume fruit juice to lose some weight, you must not consume dense juice.

Keep a Water Bottle with You

Always equip your bag with a bottle of water. Even drinking water burns calories. It is quite wrong to have cold drink or aerated drink when thirsty.

It is not proper to reduce diet to lose weight. If you wish to lose weight and decrease obesity, you have to know the balanced quantity of diet for yourself.

□

63

Eat Spicy to Lose Weight

You cannot enjoy food without spices and condiments in your food. However, are you aware that spices and condiments can help you reduce weight too?

Indian condiments such as turmeric, red chilli, black pepper and the like have a hoard of advantages to your health, and they also help to lose weight. Condiments have fewer calories as well as less fat. Let us find out if we can lose weight using spices and condiments.

- Whenever you eat sharp spicy food, the fat collected in your body starts burning and the body becomes warm.
- The rate of metabolism increases on the intake of spicy

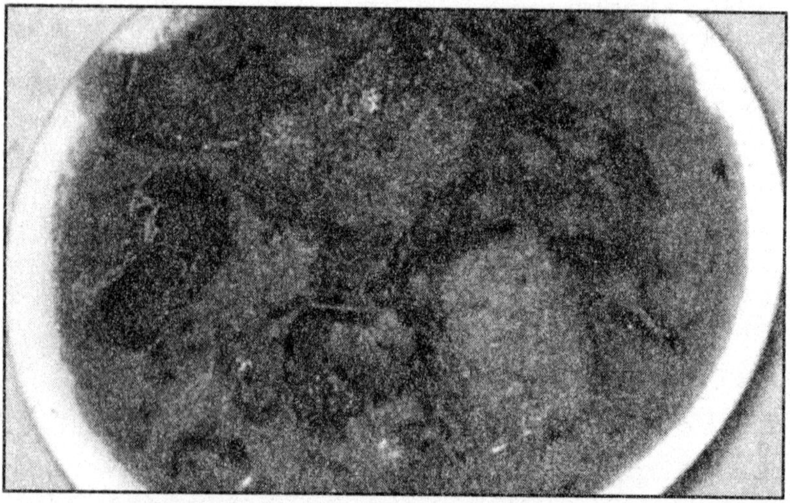

foods. In this case, your body burns energy quickly and effectively.

- Some spices, like red chilli, suppress appetite. If you use these spices, you will not feel hungry for some time. If you wish to keep your appetite under control, start using spicy food.
- If you are suffering from sinus, headache, vomiting or cough, you should start taking spicy food. They open the nasal passages, and keep you active.
- Most spices and condiments (red chilli, black pepper) contain capsosin, which makes them sharp. When you eat them, the fat collected in your body starts to burn, and your power of immunity enhances.
- Spicy food prevents the problem of constipation.

Caution is Necessary

- Spicy food can be good only when eaten in a limited quantity. Excess of spicy food can lead to several problems in the abdomen, such as ulcer, intestinal problems and bodily swelling etc.

□

64

Use Coconut Oil in Cooking

Coconut oil is easily available in every household. It not only augments taste in the food, but also helps in limiting weight. If you are aware of your diet and are always worried regarding your increasing weight, then you need to change your cooking oil. It begets the following advantages.

- Coconut oil can be digested quite easily because it contains little fatty acid, the consumption of which does not allow fat to get collected in the body.
- Triglyceride found in coconut oil enhances the rate of metabolism in the body which transforms fatty acid into energy.
- Consumption of coconut oil can also quench your

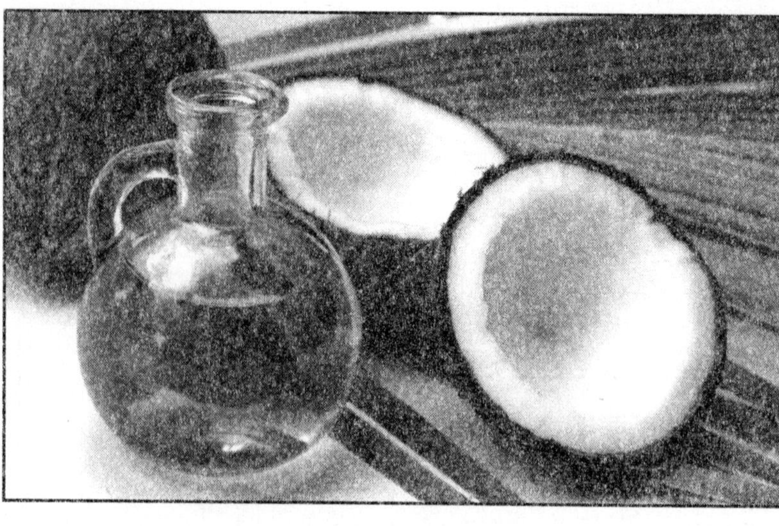

appetite that you feel frequently. This oil contains more of carbohydrates and calories, which are helpful in suppressing appetite.

- If you shift to coconut oil completely and avoid all other oils, you will be able to lose weight rather easily.
- If you wish to increase your rate of metabolism and lose weight, just mix a spoonful of oil in warm water, and drink this water before taking physical exercise. This will help you reduce weight quite quickly.
- Coconut oil slows down your digestion, which delays digestion of food and you feel less hungry. In addition, it also helps in controlling glucose in the blood.
- Candida is a type of yeast which works to increase weight, awaken hunger and augment fatigue; however, the consumption of coconut oil can help to decrease its effect.
- If you wish to take maximum advantage from coconut oil, just use unrefined or biological oil only.

□

65
Useful Points

Obesity is a disease which can create a number of several other diseases in the body. It makes a person look shabby, while he has to deprive himself of a number of foods. Therefore, it is vital that a bid to lose weight should be made as soon as possible.

- Take physical exercise or play a game regularly. Badminton, cricket, tennis, swimming, volleyball, football and many other games help to activate the body which helps to burn calories collected in fat cells. It makes the body energetic and active, while it disallows unnecessary fat to get collected in the body.
- Take training in a yoga camp. Different types of yogas are helpful in losing weight. Dhanurasana is very effective in losing fat round waist, abdomen and hips. Vajrasana helps to remove heaviness of the body. In the same manner, different other asanas help to reduce fat not necessary for the body.
- You can also adopt a number of domestic measures. Take rice starch (mand) 20 gm and mix *saindha* salt (rock salt), and consume it. Its regular daily intake helps to lose weight.
- Take 50 gm of spinach juice. Add 10 gm of lemon juice in it and drink for benefit.
- Consume 5 gm of trifala morning and evening with warm water.
- Grind zeera and pepper and have the mixture in a small amount daily morning and evening.

- Be careful about eating. Avoid fried and fatty foods. Replace them with roasted gram or puffed rice etc. Consume more of fruits and vegetables. Drink lot of water.
- Stop consuming cold drinks and chocolate. Replace aerated drinks with lemon water and buttermilk which remains a better option.
- Eat more of fat-free foods. Don't eat spicy foods. Sweet is a foe of health and slimness, so avoid it.
- Reduce the consumption of rice, tea and coffee. If you wish to eat rice, remove starch from it.

□

66

Be Creative to Lose Weight

Everybody desires to be handsome and beautiful but that requires to be slim and thin. If you wish to have this type of body, you have to make some efforts. The first thing to do for a slim, thin and shapely body is to control your diet. Control over diet does not mean decreasing the intake of food, rather it means to eat limited, sit cross-leg to eat good and nutritious food and take adequate physical exercise and work. If you make all these a regular feature of your daily life, you will not need to control your diet drastically.

When thinking of physical work to lose weight, you have to consider the following measures.

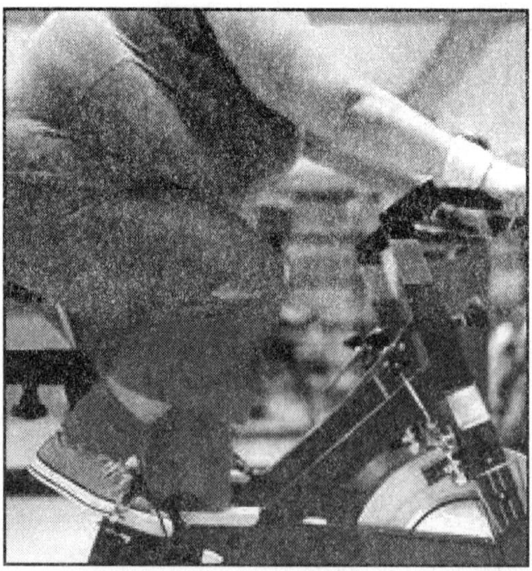

Sleep early and rise early before the sunrise. Go for a walk regularly. While walking, increase your pace gradually. Running is a good exercise but walking briskly is even more beneficial. It is good rather more beneficial for girls to skip rope.

Games and exercise are forms of physical work. When we assign all our domestic and office tasks to servants and maids, we are susceptible to two types of harms. Firstly, the work will not be done as we want it to be done. Secondly, when you have assigned your work to a helper, you are likely to stick to chair and relax and this can do nothing but expand your waist. Doing household work yourself helps to burn extra calories and keeps you healthy.

Many people are habituated of finishing their office, business or household work only to end it with a rest on the bed. This is a bad habit. Taking rest is one thing and lying on the bed all the time another. It leads to indolence, lethargy and laziness. At the same time, it slows down your digestion system. If you undertake some creative work at every time, you can keep yourself busy and your body active.

The more active you are, the more busier you are. A sound mind lives in a sound body.

Some people possess a dangerous habit of chewing all the time like a buffalo. They keep eating one thing or the other at all times and this keeps supplying the body with calories even when not needed can lead to nothing but gain in weight.

□

67
Swing and Hang

Swinging and hanging exercises and asanas are like nectar for obese people. These help to remove fat from around waist and hips and make the body active.

The spine is the foundation of the body. As a massive strong edifice cannot be built on a weak foundation so is the case with spine. A person with weak spine cannot remain strong, healthy and fit.

Yoga keeps the body fit. We need yoga to strengthen and shape our other body organs. This is true for the spine too.

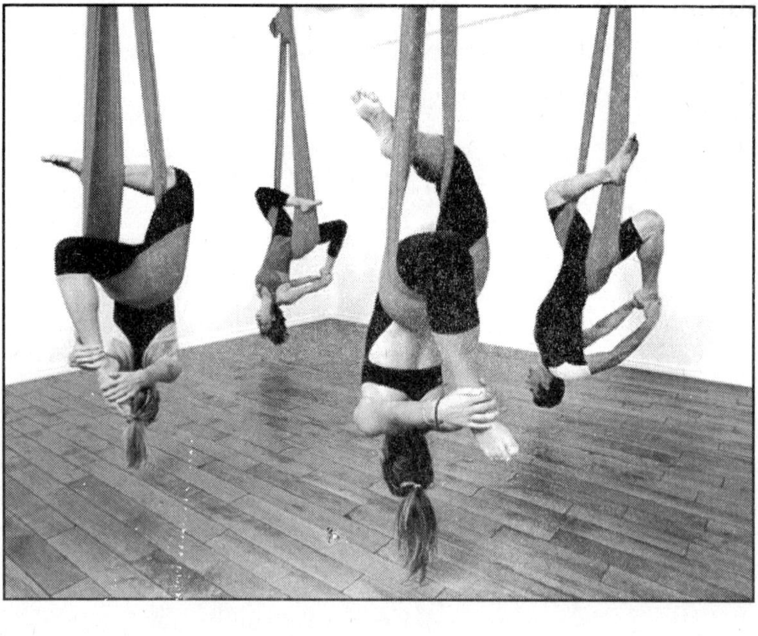

The most suitable yoga to keep the spine or backbone strong is to undertake swinging and hanging asanas. They make the spine stronger, more flexible and help the vertebrae fitter. They also help to resolve all abdominal ailments. Back muscles get a boost by these exercises.

Not only this, if you do these asanas regularly, your body becomes active and energetic. They remove fat from around your waist and hips. This is like the most effective remedy for obese people.

The good thing about these is that these asanas are very easy to do.

Method

Lie down on the ground. Fold your knees and bring them towards the chest and then hold them with arms. Now, breathe in and swing forward releasing the breath. Breathe in while swinging backward.

Keep your head safe from knocking down and try to swing so far forward as to sit on the feet.

Caution

This process exercises all joints and vertebrae of the spine as you swing forward and backward on the backbone. Those suffering from backache should avoid this exercise. When you do this in the morning hours, this infuses energy in your body.

□

68

Eat Breakfast to Lose Weight

The most important meal of the day is the morning meal or breakfast. It is believed that if you eat full, you will keep healthy. It will also keep you away from fast foods and junk foods as you won't feel hungry. Come, let us find out how breakfast can help you lose weight.

- Normally those who eat one-half of their daily diet in the morning, they do not gain weight as compared with those who don't do this.

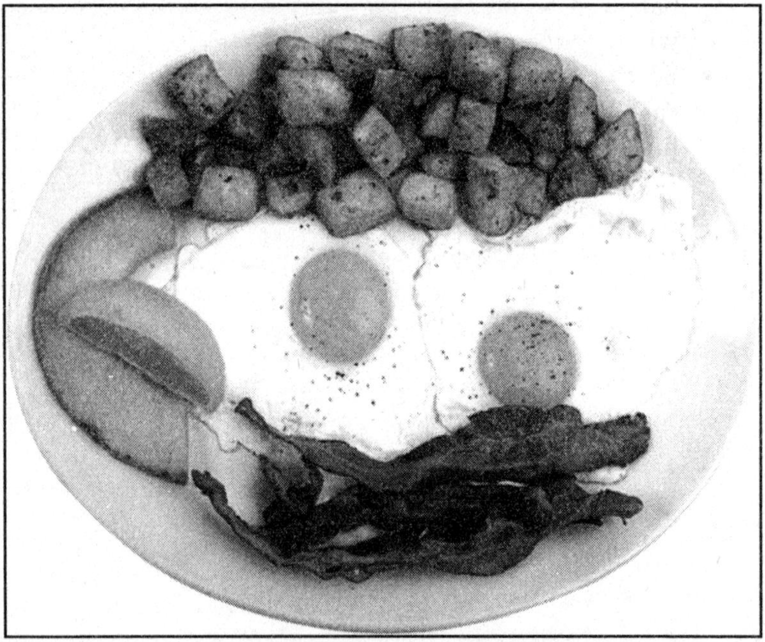

- The people who don't eat breakfast keep feeling hungry and they keep laying their hands over some or the other snacks, biscuits and salted foods during the daytime and this can do nothing but increase weight.
- Not only those who avoid breakfast, but those who eat light breakfast or don't eat it properly too, invite obesity on a platter also.
- If you consume 1,200-1,300 calories in breakfast, you will not need any additional calories round the day. You can follow this up with 400 calories in lunch and another 300 calories in dinner; and this will keep you light and fit.
- Generally, a fit person requires 2,000 calories throughout the day but the need for calories depends on your lifestyle and working style.
- If you prefer diet with fewer carbohydrates, it would certainly lead to less weight, but you cannot keep healthy for long and it will make you gain weight once again after some time. On the other hand, if you take a balanced breakfast in the morning hours, your weight will come down for all the times to come.
- Scientists are of the view that consuming fewer carbohydrates decreases weight but it causes more hunger, which slows down digestion.

□

69
Dance to Lose Weight

The people afflicted by obesity, who do not like to do yoga or workout in a gym, can well lose weight by dancing. Dancing is a recreational activity together with being a good exercise for the body. It keeps the body healthy if you dance everyday. It also has a positive impact on the mind, making you happy and delighted. Those who dance regularly are not inflicted by the problem of obesity. If obese people dance daily,

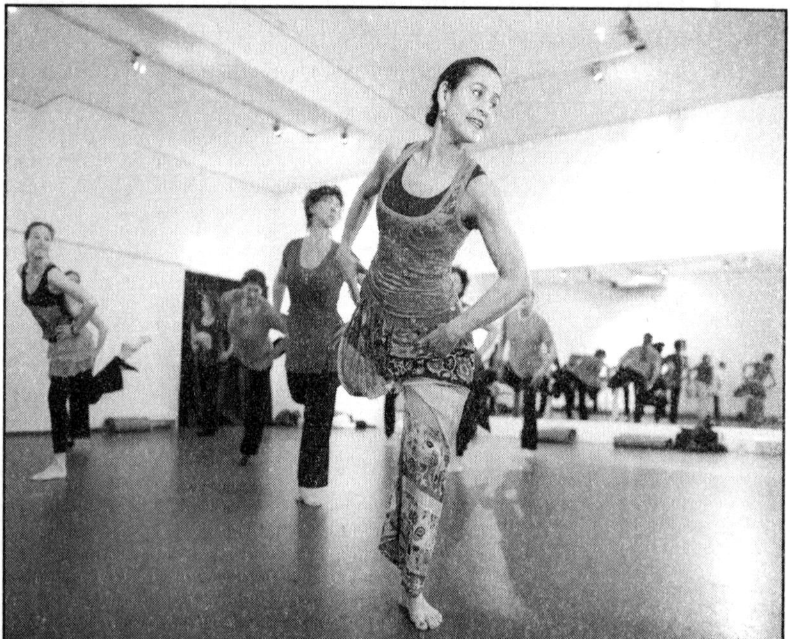

they can overcome the problem of obesity. Dancing for at least 5 minutes helps you burn away 30 calories. The people who begin dancing at a small age are able to keep their weight under control.

A study has revealed the fact that the people who dance from a small age are able to keep their weight under control, while not having to face any problems like stress or depression.

If you are a victim of obesity and do not like to do yoga or work hard in a gym then dancing can be a good option for you. Come, let us find out how we can lose weight while dancing.

- Dance is done for fun and celebration but this helps to burn off extra fat from the body and keep your obesity under control.
- Start dancing to your favourite song. You can dance to the tune of your music system in the morning. You can do it in your room or on the roof.
- Salsa and belly dance help to finish off fat round the waist.
- Hip-hop and salsa dances help to burn out large number of calories.
- Those who cannot dance at a swift rate and they dance at a slow pace, they also benefit from dancing as they too burn calories at a larger rate.
- Do aerobics to the tune of a song at home. It is also a type of dance.
- Different steps of aerobics help to reduce fat from different parts of the body.
- Dancing exercises both hands and feet, as well as all other organs of the body. The blood starts to flow rapidly in the body.
- Dancing strengthens the muscles.
- Dancing for half an hour a day can help reduce 5-10 kg of body weight in a month.

□

70

Beverages for Weight Loss

Liquids should be taken abundantly in order to keep healthy and active but beverages should not be harmful to the body. Beverages like juice, soup, lemon water, water and the like can help you overcome the problem of obesity effectively. The beverages containing minimal sugar are very good, so are the lemon beverages, carbonate beverages, etc.

Come, let us find out how we can lose weight by the consumption of beverages.

- People tend to think that fruit juice can gain weight but

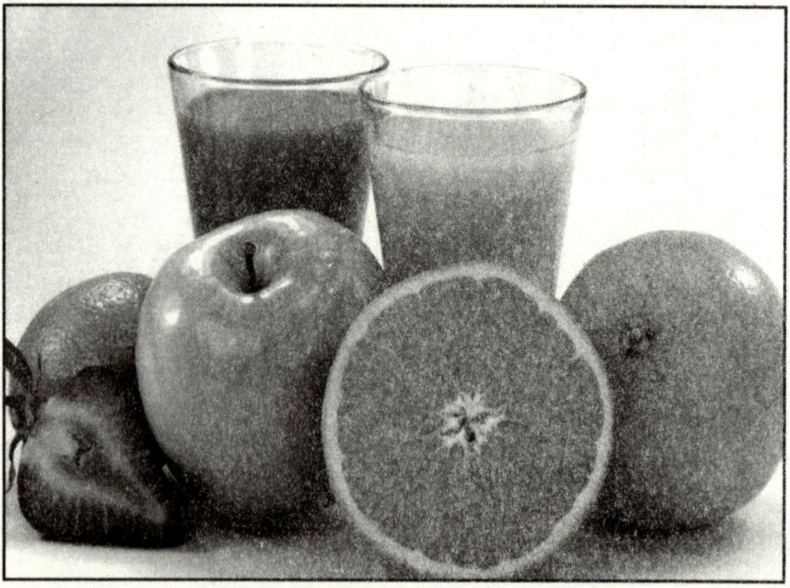

a research has revealed that it is helpful in losing weight if it is fully pure without sugar having been mixed in it.

- Of all beverages, fruit juices are the most beneficial. As a matter of fact, those who drink fruit juices do not get fat; on the other hand, fruit juices help to supply their body with vitamin C, potassium, magnesium, foliate, iron and other nutrients.
- Beverages like soft drinks and cold (aerated) drinks cause an increase in weight; while milk, water, coconut water, juice, etc. are helpful in reducing weight.
- Not only fruit juices but water can also contribute to losing weight quite easily. For this, you have to drink two glasses of water before meals, which will make you feel less hungry stopping you short of your appetite.
- Normally, tea helps to lose weight too. It also keeps you active and agile but it should be without milk. In fact, all the benefits of tea are done away with as soon as milk is added to it. Besides, it also does away with the protein supplied by milk.
- You can take black tea, green tea, lemon tea and the like to lose weight. This will protect you from the negative effect and you can keep your weight under control too.
- Having lemon water with honey in the morning can help to reduce weight.
- You can also consume juice of green vegetables as beverages. It will help you decrease weight quite easily.

□

71

Quit Sweets to Lose Weight

The foremost principle of losing weight is to keep off sweets. However, it is not an easy a task to refuse your favourite sweet or for that matter chocolate, when you have it right before your eyes. Often we fail to understand how we can overcome the desire to eat sweet.

The problem is based on our ignorance how much sugar we should consume. It is an extremely important fact that more sugar in our diet burns less energy and fuel. It leaves a

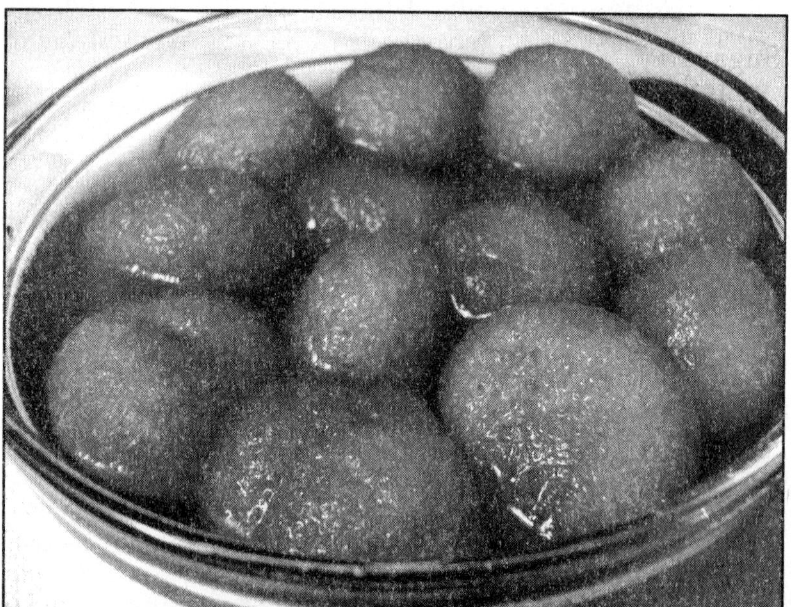

negative impact when consumed in excessive quantity. It also increases weight, while giving an open invitation to some ailments like diabetes.

Estimate Your Habits

Pay attention to your eating habits. Do you have sweet before or after lunch? What time of the day compels you to have sweet? These factors might look insignificant to you, yet you can bring about a change in them in order to keep healthy and fit. If you estimate your habits, you will be able to find out that you are taking extra sugar. This will make you replace sweet with other healthy foods. For example, if you have sweet in breakfast, you should replace it with some other food which can give you energy.

Say 'No' to Sugar

Set your 'no sugar' goal. Keep reminding yourself that you have set this goal in your own interest. You may have to work hard to achieve this goal. You can achieve this goal by bringing about a change in your diet.

Sugar-free Beverages

If you love to have tea or coffee, make them sugar-less. You can instead use honey or syrup in beverages.

Say 'No' to Sweets

It would be better for you to give up the habit of eating sweet in meals. If you are habitual of having sweets after meals, reduce these instances to thrice a week in the beginning; at the same time, limit the quantity of sweet every time.

□

72

Swim to Lose Weight

You can swim for half an hour to burn 400 calories. Swimming is a wholesome exercise than yoga and workout. Swift swimming comforts the body because the body moves in the water. It helps to augment blood circulation, which helps to relieve headache and stress.

Advantages of Swimming

- You have to put in 12 times more hard work as compared to floor exercise because there is 12 times more resistance in water.
- Swimming can help to control obesity. Swimming for 30 minutes can burn your 400 calories.

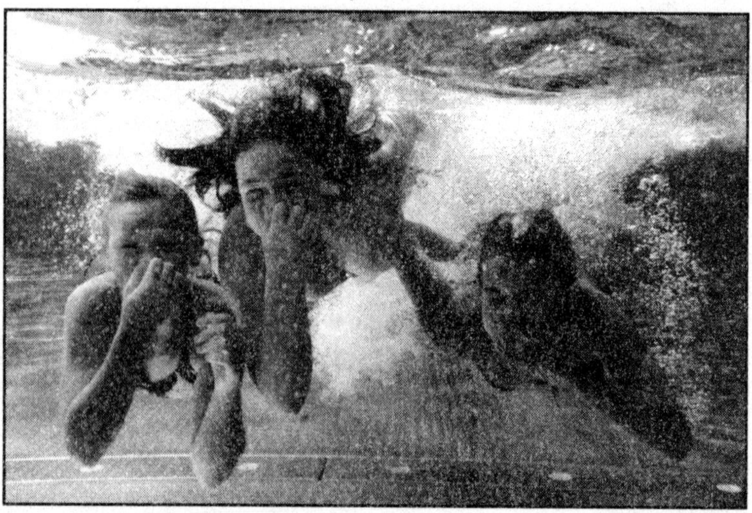

- Swimming is a good heart exercise which is more advantageous in comparison to other exercises because the body moves through the water.
- Swimming also controls blood pressure and blood cholesterol.
- Swimming causes swift respiration which strengthens lungs. It also reduces the instances of stroke, heart attack and diabetes.
- Swimming daily can help to make the body and joints flexible which boosts energy and strengthens muscles.

Different Activities in Swimming

1. **Front Stroke:** In front stroke, you swim to the front, in which both arms rotate from below, while both legs move in turn.
2. **Breast Stroke:** In this stroke, both arms move together in the beginning and both legs take over the movement.
3. **Back Stroke:** This is swimming on the back.
4. **Butterfly Stroke:** In this type of swimming, the thorax, arms and head protrude out of water first and then both legs move together.

□

73
Some Useful Tips

- Whenever you go to market to buy things, make sure to find out the level of fat and sugar. Make sure, in particular, to avoid the use of saturated fats.
- If you consume more fatty products, replace them with low fatty products. In this way, you can reduce the quantity of fat in your diet. This helps you overcome your attraction towards fats gradually.
- When you sit to eat, don't take variety of items at a time. Avoid eating different items uncontrollably. Eat only those things which you can digest easily. When you are hungry and sit to eat, determine in advance what you are going to eat and what impact it will have on your body. If you don't do this, your mind can revolt as soon as you open the refrigerator and find your favourite dishes right before your eyes, making you eager to eat them.
- Don't kill your mind. If you wish to take chocolate, take it but limit yourself to a small piece. If you avoid chocolate completely, you may shift to banana and then to biscuit, and finally you will revert to chocolate more in a revengeful manner.
- Never look for alternatives for meals. Never find excuse for eating fast foods or junk foods because of convenience or lack of time. As and when it may be possible, take time out of your busy schedule in order to have the right and balanced diet. Light food, when taken as a replacement for regular meal can neither get you satisfaction nor can it give

you nutrition. Moreover, this will make you eat more heavily in the next meal, and this is a possible cause of weight gain.

- Like other activities and requirements of your life, adopt a planned manner in diet too. When you set out for office from home, you should have your home-cooked lunch with you. Your lunch box should also contain some fruit or snack, so that you don't have to opt for some unhealthy foods if you need to chew something.
- If you are really serious about your weight, you have to keep an eye over it. Keep watching what you are eating and what is its impact on you. Weigh yourself from time to time and bring about a change in your exercise regimen accordingly.

□

74

What Balanced Diet Is

Many people are aware of the contribution of balanced diet in good health but they possess a number of misconceptions regarding what balanced diet is.

Some people are prone to think that stomach-ful of food makes a balanced diet, while others can think that expensive food is a balanced diet. But the fact is far from this. It is not at all necessary for a balanced diet to be stomach-ful, expensive or tasty. Foods in limited quantity, cheap in price and ordinary in look too can make up a balanced diet.

As you might know that the necessary nutrients of food are proteins, carbohydrates, fats, minerals, salts, vitamins and

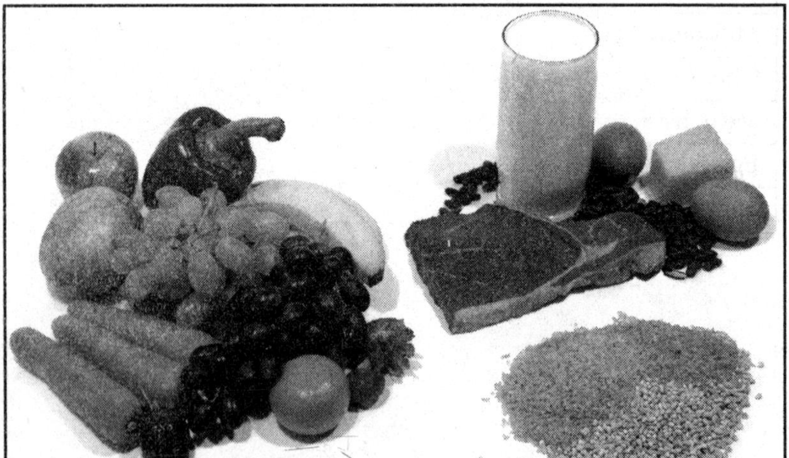

water etc. These nutrients play different roles as some of them supply energy to the body, while others are necessary for building of the body; and still others contribute in controlling physiological processes in the body so as to keep it healthy.

By a balanced diet is meant to receive all those nutrients in proper ratio and quantity.

Thus, a balanced diet supplies the body with all needs pertaining to nutrition.

If you want to have a normal body, it is essential for you to know about a balanced diet. It will also be helpful in reducing your obesity and losing weight. Before the process of your obesity sets in, you should plan for your balanced diet in accordance with the following diet chart.

Food Items	*Non-vegetarian Food Items (in gm)*	*Vegetarian Food Items (in gm)*
Grains	350	350
Pulses	60	75
Green leafy vegetables	125	125
Other vegetables	75	75
Fruits	30	30
Milk and milk products	125	200
Ghee or oil	35	30
Meat, fish	30	–
Eggs	30	–
Sugar, jaggery	30	30

□

75

Planned Exercise and Lose Weight

The body is made for activity. In the changing lifestyle of modern times, the means of comfort and luxury have become manifold to the extent that the body is unable to find some work that requires hard work. Now, more importance is attached to the mental work as compared to the physical work. Often, people are engaged in mental work still they keep taking a diet which is fit only for physical work. As a result, they are not able to consume the calories received from such a diet. Soon they find themselves overweight and obese and become susceptible to a number of ailments. Thus, we can see how vital physical activity is for good health.

You will find many people not eating much but they are still obese. It is normal to wonder about it. In fact, they are the

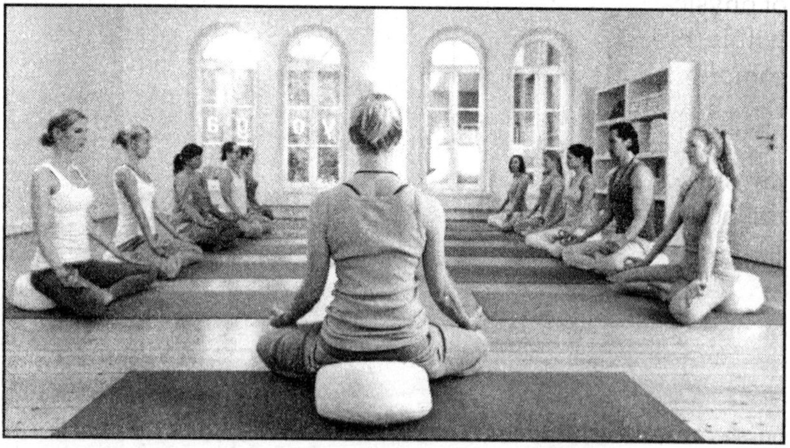

people who are little active physically due to which their body spends little energy. Little consumption of energy in the body is the chief cause of obesity in the body. If a person consumes a diet in comparison with the involved physical activity, he will never get fat.

The modern era has introduced machines in every sphere of life and the comfort and inactivity resulting from these machines has diminished physical activity of man. In such a situation, a person is bound to take physical exercise in order to remain physically active.

In a research conducted over a period of one year, men and women were placed in two different groups in order to ascertain the level of obesity experienced by them. In this study, the subjects in a group were given only controlled diet as per the dietary plans in order to achieve loss of weight; while on the subjects in the other group, effort was made to introduce physical workout as well as dieting. After some time, it was observed that the people undergoing dieting as well as physical exercise lost more weight as compared with those who were put only on a dietary plan. This study infers that exercise plays a vital role in losing weight and decreasing obesity.

As the body grows unshapely and shabby due to obesity, a person might feel inferiority complex. Often, he is hesitant and unable to mix up with other people around and this limits his activity within himself. He also keeps postponing the matter of physical exercise due to this hesitation. As he remains limited within himself, he is prone to cultivate a sense of inferiority complex, leading to stress. He then takes part in social activities. Loss in weight also infuses new confidence in him.

In conclusion, we can say that exercise helps all physiological systems work properly by which all organs of the body start functioning normally and effectively.

□

76

Exercise Intensifies Calorie Consumption

The body requires energy to do any activity. Depending on size or height, two different people will require different amounts of calories to undertake the same kind of activity. A person consumes few calories during sleep. When you sit idly, about 1 calorie is spent in 1 minute. Remember, you cannot gain weight in a single day nor can it be decreased in a single day. If you burn 3,500 calories, you can decrease your weight by half a kilo. So much of calorie consumption cannot reach that level all of a sudden. Exercise helps to boost up this energy consumption.

Exercise Shapes the Body

An unshapely person looks shabby, often fun is cut at the person. Regular exercise helps to tone up the body while helping to lose weight. It also tones up muscular tissues leading to a shapely body. If obesity is decreasing quickly, it lowers the level of fat in the body; however, the skin cannot shrink in that proportion. Therefore, there may be wrinkles in different parts of the body. If you take exercise, you can overcome this problem of wrinkles.

Exercise Controls Appetite

When you take up light exercise, your blood circulation improves. When the blood circulates at a lower rate in the digestive system, you feel less of appetite. You can certainly feel thirsty. Taking up light exercise a little before lunch can help you keep your weight under control. You will find satisfaction with even little food. Taking excessive and varied exercises bring down the level of sugar in the blood, which makes you feel hungry. Therefore, it is advisable to undertake light exercise before meals.

Exercise Stabilises the Level of Obesity

Losing weight is a simpler thing to do but it is quite a difficult task to maintain the reduced level of weight. Once you have lost weight, you have to keep taking physical exercises and work so that you don't revert to your previous obese condition. Thus, exercise helps you maintain the level of obesity. □

77

Lose Weight with Good Carbohydrates

In a study conducted at Harvard, about 75,000 women were included as the subjects. Of these, the subjects who took high fibre food in both meals, they were found less susceptible to weight gain by 50 percent, when compared with women who consumed refined carbohydrates (harmful or bad carbohydrates). The research also concluded that during the digestion process, good beneficial fibre carbohydrates help to consume more calories, and such a diet causes the stomach to fill up rather quickly. If you consume high fibre bread, cereals, pasta and rice, it controls the quantity of insulin and this helps in controlling weight and losing fat. It is evident that a diet loaded with good carbohydrates can help to lose weight beneficially.

Most vegetables (other than white potato and corn), fruits (not fruit juice), beans, dry fruits, grains and chapattis have a lower glycemic index. They can be included in the category of good carbohydrates. Your body changes good carbohydrate food into glucose which is rectified in the intestine at a slow rate which then blends with the blood vessels.

As glucose is absorbed slowly, the amount of insulin produced in the stomach too is kept under control. This balanced level of insulin supplies glucose to the blood vessels slowly so that energy can be produced. In other words, due to absence of abnormal amount of insulin and glucose, extra fat cannot be collected in the blood vessels and weight cannot be gained. In the absence of any variation in the level of glucose or insulin, a person does not feel hungry abnormally and he is saved from consuming bad carbohydrates.

While implementing the scheme for weight loss, taking good carbohydrate-rich diet can help a lot. Such a diet contains limited quantity of fat and calories.

In the following good carbohydrate foods, the glycemic index is lower:

1. Most vegetables other than corn and white potato.
2. Most fruits (juice not included).
3. Beans (you will find fibre, protein, vitamins, minerals and other nutrients in them).
4. Whole grains.

□

78
Bad Carbohydrates

There is no evidence to prove that in the process of weight loss there is more contribution of low-carbohydrate diet as compared to low-fat diet. Low-carbohydrate diet can bring down the weight in the initial phase but in 90 percent cases, the weight drastically increases when people give up boring fat-rich and protein-rich foods. In most cases, such people gain weight many a times even 20 percent more weight than before.

The carbohydrates consumed by you are changed by the body into glucose, which is used by the body cells as fuel. When the particles of glucose enter the blood vessels, the stomach produces insulin and asks the cells to absorb glucose. When cells (skin, internal organs, tissues, muscles, fats and others) have absorbed glucose, the level of insulin returns to its normal level.

The distinction between good and bad carbohydrates can be understood by the fact how quickly carbohydrate-rich food changes into glucose and gets absorbed in blood vessels. It is called glycemic index. The diet with a higher glycemic index is considered to fall in the category of bad or harmful carbohydrates.

A carbohydrate-rich diet with higher glycemic index changes carbohydrates into sugar in the intestines and then supplies it to the blood vessels. As blood sugar shoots up rapidly, the insulin produced by the stomach too shoots up. Due to an increase in the level of insulin, the level of blood sugar goes down because the body tissues and brain feel the need for fuel.

In such a situation, the brain transmits signals for appetite, and a person is motivated to eat something. Calorie consumption is increased due to unbalanced levels of glucose and insulin, leading to weight gain in the body.

□

79

Know the Value of Calorie

There is much talk of limited carbohydrate diet in market and media. It is being advertised through such products as bread, cake etc. that weight can be lowered using such low-carbohydrate diet. Falling in this trap, people are prone to consume lot of calories. Such an unhealthy diet contains lot of fat, which supplies the body with lot of calories. Keep in mind that you consume 9 calories with each gm of fat, while there are 4 calories in a gm of carbohydrate or protein. The proportion between the consumption of calories and the burning of calories in exercise will decide whether you will get slim or obese.

An American Institution, The National Academy of Sciences and Medicine has said in its report on diet in 2002, that we obtain 65 percent of our calories from carbohydrates. That means, 520 calories out of a daily intake of 1,200 calories are taken from carbohydrates.

Carbohydrates transform into glucose which is a source of fuel to the body and brain. If you stop taking carbohydrates, your muscles and liver will experience the lack of carbohydrates and your body will start producing glucose from protein which is an insufficient method of producing energy. Such a case leads to fatigue, depression, mineral imbalance and the loss of protein in the body. As has been discussed before, this type of imbalance leads to a pressure on the kidneys, liver and other intrinsic organs and if one continues with the same kind of diet, these organs can be irreparably harmed.

The body feels the need for carbohydrates to work well. However, the body does not need extra calories in the form of refined sugar nor does it require additional amount of starch and fat. Therefore, when you don't include such food items, such calories are not included in your diet and you find yourself in a better position of losing weight.

□

80

What Calorie Is

We can see that the dietary requirement of a person undertaking physical work is different from a person doing desk work. In the same manner, the dietary needs of children, adolescents and women are quite varied. The dietary needs for the body are calculated by calorie.

As we use the measurement in form of metre for length or height, or kilogram for weight, the energy supplied to the body through food is measured by calorie. Thus, calorie is a unit of energy. The amount of heat or energy needed to heat 1 litre of water to 1 degree centigrade is called 1 calorie.

All the activities we undertake everyday require energy consumption. Energy is consumed in our sitting and standing, working, chewing food, walking, running and the like. The body also burns calories in all activities, small or big.

A person with normal body weight consumes different number of calories in different activities per hour, which can be enumerated as follows:

- In sleep : 50–55
- Lying : 55–70
- Sitting at rest : 75–80
- Standing at rest : 85–90
- Writing : 100–105
- Typing or like work : 110
- Doing hand work : 130
- Doing light work : 135
- Washing clothes by hand : 140

- Walking at a normal pace : 190
- Walking briskly : 235
- Running : 395
- Doing physical work : 230
- Doing hard work : 310

□

81

Calorie Value of Food

We consume different types of food items in our daily life. Each food item supplies us with energy in varying amount. There is no food which lacks calorie altogether. Some foods items have calories in abundant quantity, while others may be deficient in it. By calorie value of a food item is meant the energy or calorie obtained from it. In the table given below is enumerated the value of calorie present in different necessary elements present in food items:

Calorie Value of Nutrients in Food

Nutrients	*Calorie Value*
1 gm protein	4
1 gm carbohydrate	4
1 gm fat	9
Vitamins, minerals, salts,	0
water and fibre	

Required Calories as per Age

Age Group	*Number of Calories*
1–2 years	700
2–3 years	950
3–5 years	1,200
5–7 years	1,680

7–9 years	1,900
9–11 years	2,200
11–14 years	2,400
A normally healthy person	2,500–2,800
A hard working person	3,000–3,200
A heavy hard working person	2,500–2,800
Lactating mother	3,000–3,200

1200 Calorie/Day Diet Plan Vegetarian

Food Groups	*Quantity*	*Domestic Measurement*
Milk (toned or without cream)	350 ml	1 ½ cup
Grains	125 gm	5 chapattis
Pulses	30 gm	1 medium bowl
Green leafy	350 gm	3 medium bowls
vegetables	100 gm	1 medium bowl
Other vegetables		
Fruits	250 gm	2 medium
Cooking oil	10 ml	2 tea spoonful
Sugar	Nil	Nil
Nuts	7 gm	5 almond or 2 half walnuts

Morning	Tea (with milk) 1 cup (20 calories) Nuts (consumption of half) (30 calories) (5 almonds or 2 half walnuts)	**50 calories**
Breakfast	1 small bowl cooked dalia/ wheat flakes/1 idli/ 1 slice bread (veg sandwich) 85 calories Milk (toned) 1 glass	**215 calories**

	(130 calories) or 1 boiled egg (100 calories)	
Mid-morning	Fruits 1 medium size apple/ orange/guava/pear (60 calories)	**60 calories**
Lunch	Salad 1 medium bowl (20 calories) Green leafy vegetables 1 small bowl (50 calories) Other vegetables 1 small bowl (70 calories) Curd/vegetable raita 1 small bowl (130 calories) 2 medium chapattis or 1 medium bowl rice (170 calories)	**440 calories**
Evening Tea	Fresh lime/tea with milk 1 cup (20 calories) Fruits 1 medium 2 medium size (60 calories)	**80 calories**
Dinner	Salad 1 medium plate (20 calories) Green leafy vegetables 1 medium bowl (75 calories) Dal (pulse) whole 1 medium bowl (150 calories), or 1 medium chapatti (85 calories)	**330 calories**

1400 Calorie/Day Diet Plan Vegetarian

Food Groups	*Quantity*	*Domestic Measurement*
Milk (toned)	450 ml	1½ medium glass
Grains	125 gm	5 chapattis
Pulses	60 gm	2 medium bowls
Green leafy	350 gm	3 medium bowls
Vegetables	10 gm	1 medium bowl

Other vegetables	250 gm	2 medium size
Fruits	15 ml	3 tea spoons
Cooking oil	Nil	Nil
SugarNuts	7 gm	5 almonds or 2 half walnuts

Morning
Tea with milk 1 cup (20 calories)
Nuts (one-half) (30 calories)
5 almonds or 2 half walnuts **50 calories**

Breakfast
1 medium bowl cooked dalia/
wheat flakes/vegetable poha/
vegetable upama/
2 idlis/1 small dosa/
2 slice bread (veg sandwich)/ **350 calories**
1 vegetable (spinach)/
1 stuffed roti (220 calories)
Milk 1 glass (130 calories)
or boiled egg (100 calories)

Mid-morning
Fruits 1 medium size apple/
orange/guava/pear 60 calories
60 calories

Lunch
Salad 1 medium bowl
(20 calories)
Green leafy vegetables 1 bowl
(50 calories)
Pulses (whole) 1 medium bowl)
(150 calories)
Curd/vegetable raita
1 small bowl (130 calories) **520 calories**
2 medium chapattis/2 medium
bowl rice (170 calories)

Evening Tea
Tea with milk 1 cup
(20 calories)

	Fruits 1 medium size (60 calories)	**80 calories**
Dinner	Salad 1 medium bowl (20 calories) Mixed veg 1 medium bowl (70 calories), or 1 medium chapatti (85 calories)	**325 calories**

1600 Calorie/Day Diet Plan Vegetarian

Food Groups	*Quantity*	*Domestic Measurement*
Milk (toned)	500 ml	2 medium glasses
Grains	150 gm	6 times
Pulses	60 gm	2 medium bowls
Green leafy vegetables	350 gm	3 medium bowls
Other vegetables	100 gm	1 medium bowl
Fruits	250 gm	2 medium size
Cooking oil	15 ml	3 tea spoon
Sugar	Nil	Nil
Nuts	7 gm	7 almonds or 4 half walnuts

Morning	Tea with milk 1 cup (20 calories) Nuts (consumption of half) (30 calories) (5 almonds or 2 half walnuts)	**50 calories**
Breakfast	1 medium bow l cooked dalia or wheat flakes/veg poha/ veg upama/2 idlis/ 1 small dosa/2 slice bread (veg sandwich)/1 veg (spinach) /stuffed roti (220 calories) Milk (toned) 1 glass (130 calories), or 1 boiled egg (100 calories)	**350 calories**

Mid-morning	Fruit 1 medium size (apple/orange/guava/pear) (60 calories)	**60 calories**
Lunch	Salad 1 medium plate (20 calories) Green leafy vegetables 2 medium bowls (100 calories) Dal (whole) 1 medium bowl (150 calories) Curd/veg raita 1 small bowl (130 calories) 2 medium chapattis/ 2 medium bowl rice (170 calories)	**570 calories**
Evening Tea	Tea with milk 1 cup (20 calories) Fruit 1 medium (60 calories)	**80 calories**
Dinner	Salad 1 medium plate (20 calories) Mixed vegetables 1 medium bowl (70 calories) Dal 1 medium bowl (150 calories), or 2 medium chapattis (170 calories)	**410 calories**

1800 Calorie/Day Diet Plan Vegetarian

Food Groups	*Quantity*	*Domestic Measurement*
Milk (toned)	750 ml	3 medium glasses
Grains	200 gm	7–8 servings
Dals	60 gm	2 medium bowls
Green leafy vegetables	300 gm	3 medium bowls
Other vegetables	200 gm	2 medium bowls

Fruits	300 gm	3 medium size
Cooking oil	15–20 ml	3–4 tea spoon
Sugar	Nil	Nil
Nuts	12 gm	8 almonds or 4 half walnuts

Morning Tea with milk 1 cup (20 calories)
2 Marie biscuits (30 calories) **50 calories**

Breakfast Vegetable (spinach)
stuffed chapattis/2 medium bowl
cooked dalia/wheat flakes/
veg poha/veg upama/2-3 idlis/
2 small dosas/2 slice bread
(veg sandwich) (220 calories) **380 calories**
Milk (toned) 1 glass (130 calories)
Nuts (consumption of half)
7 almonds or 4 half walnuts
(30 calories)

Mid-morning Fruits 1 medium size apple/
orange/guava/pear
(60 calories) **60 calories**

Lunch Salad 1 medium plate
(20 calories)
Green leafy vegetables
2 medium bowls (100 calories)
Das (whole) 1 medium bowl
(150 calories) **655 calories**
Curd/veg raita 1 small bowl
(130 calories)
Chapattis/idli/plain dosa
3 medium size (225 calories), or
2 medium bowls of rice +
1 chapatti (225 calories)

Evening Tea Tea/milk/fresh lime 1 cup

	(without sugar) (20 calories) Roasted gram dal mixture 1 bowl (50 calories) or Fruit 1 medium size (60 calories)	**70 calories**
Dinner	Salad 1 medium plate (20 calories) Mixed vegetables 1 medium bowl (100 calories) Dal 1 medium bowl (150 calories), or Chicken/fish with gravy 2 small pieces (150 calories) 2 medium chapattis + 1 medium bowl rice (225 calories) Fruit curd 1 small bowl (100 calories)	**625 calories**

□

82

Dietary Recommendations

- Have meals at fixed time of the day. Don't force food in when not hungry.
- Always have fresh, clean and warm food.
- Always eat at a clean and tranquil place.
- Sit down to eat. It is easy to guess if you have a full stomach.
- Eat delightfully. If you are inflicted with worry, anxiety, stress, tension, anger, jealousy, playfulness or the like emotions then you will not be able to eat well. In such situations a person is in wont of eating more than or less than necessary.
- Never force in food. If you don't like eating, just give it up. Never force children to keep eating.
- Don't talk while eating. Eat attentively. Don't watch television while eating. Many people are prone to leave eating or eat more than required while watching television.
- Drink little water while eating. If you keep drinking water during meals, the necessary pores in the food canal become weak, leading to improper digestion.
- Don't eat food soon after hard work or workout.
- Chew well slowly and for long. Some people chew less and swallow more. The more you chew food, the easier becomes the digestion process. If you eat in a hurry, you are inclined to eat more.
- Don't eat food in a hurry or while walking around.

- It is good to have a little rest after lunch, while it is advisable to go for a small walk after dinner.
- Don't eat anything for three hours after meals. Normally, there should be an interval of at least 5 hours between two meals.
- It is good to have one or two glasses of water in the morning after you leave bed. It makes the digestion system healthy.
- If you are suffering from a problem like constipation or acidity, it would be better to give up one meal or fast for sometime.

□

83
Reliable Diet Control Scheme

Most people who wish to reduce their obesity, immediately think of controlling their diet. Most of the obese people are prone to think of controlling their obesity by reducing their diet.

Diet control can certainly lead to reduce obesity, but this control will have to be continued for a long period of time i.e. continuously. Once you have lost weight, you must not resume your previous dietary regimen else, you will certainly regain the previous obese condition.

An important factor that is linked with dietary regimen is exercise. Only dieting cannot lead to long-term weight loss. Exercise is necessary for this purpose. Thus, weight loss is contributed by dietary control as well as physical exercise. Therefore, both these should be brought into practice simultaneously.

There are different ways by which dietary control can be applied. Dieticians are yet to form a uniform opinion regarding this; but it should be kept in mind that crash or fad dieting methods are very harmful and all dieticians agree with this view. Normal and reliable dietary control scheme alone can lead you to your coveted goal. This scheme is fully safe as well as effective.

Extra quantity of food taken collects in the body in the form of fat. Supposedly, you consume food amounting to 2,500 calories while you are able to spend only 2,000 calories in all the daily activities put together. In this case, the remaining amount of 500 calories will get collected in your body in the form of fat. On the other hand, if you consume 1,000 calories, the additional requirement of 1,000 calories will be spent from the extra fat stored in the body.

Thus, the fat stored in the body keeps changing into energy to be spent, resulting into the diminished level of fat in the body, and with this, the body weight too goes down. If normal dieting leads to consumption of 500 fewer calories per day, it will help you lose weight by half a kilo in a week. This dietary control regimen is completely safe and its positive effect can be perceived directly too.

In fact, a reliable dietary control is the one in which the amount of energy is systematically and gradually reduced. It should bring down the body weight 250 gm to 500 gm a week. You need to bring about a change in your lifestyle in order to implement a good dietary control regimen.

A controlled diet should provide your body with all essential elements in sufficient measure. This scheme should not be expensive too, so that you can continue with it regularly and continuously. Together with this scheme, you must continue with your exercise and yoga regimen too.

□

84

Controlled Diet Scheme-1

Morning

Tea without sugar, or plain or lemon water.

Morning Breakfast

1 bowl toned milk, two thin bread slices or one bowl wheat dalia.

Lunch

Rice or Chapattis – 4 thin and without ghee
Vegetables – as needed
Dal (pulse) – about one bowl
Curd – about 150 gm
Meat or fish – about 100 gm
Paneer (domestic cheese) – 60 gm

Evening Breakfast

Fruit juice – without sugar
Tea/Coffee – without sugar
Any fruit – not more than one/two

Dinner

Chapattis – 4 without ghee thin ones
vegetable – as needed
Dal – about 1 bowl

Salad	– as much as possible
Green leafy vegetables	– as needed
Pickle	– little or not at all
Paneer	– 60 gm

□

85

Controlled Diet Scheme-2

Morning on Leaving Bed

Tea	–	skimmed milk and without sugar
or plain lemon water	–	1 glass

Morning Breakfast

Fruit	–	anyone, but not more than one
Milk without cream	–	1 glass
Or egg	–	not more than one
Tea	–	without sugar

Lunch

Rice	–	boiled and unpolished 80 gm
vegetable	–	as required
Salad	–	as much as possible
Curd	–	about 100 gm
Meat or fish	–	about 100 gm

Evening Breakfast

Milk skimmed	–	1 small glass
Tea or coffee	–	without sugar
Or fruit	–	anyone

Dinner

Chapattis	–	without ghee and thin ones 4
Vegetables	–	as required
Salad	–	as much as possible
Dal from sprouts	–	1 bowl
Or meat	–	about 60 gm

□

86

Controlled Diet Scheme-3

Morning on Leaving Bed

Tea	– skimmed milk and without sugar
Or, fruit juice	– without sugar 1 glass

Morning Breakfast

Bread	– 2 slices
Tea	– skimmed milk and without sugar
Egg	– one
Or, milk skimmed	– 1 glass

Lunch

Chapattis	– thin ones without ghee 4
Or, rice	– about 80 gm
Dal	– about 60 gm
Vegetable	– about 30 gm
Salad	– as much as possible

Evening Breakfast

Tea	– without sugar skimmed milk
Or, Dal soup	– about 30 gm
Fruit	– anyone

Dinner

Chapattis	–	without ghee thin ones 4
Veg (beans or cabbage)	–	about 50 gm
Salad (onion, tomato, carrot)	–	as much as possible
Green leafy vegetable	–	about 40 gm
Or, paneer	–	about 30 gm

□

87
Controlled Diet Scheme-4

Morning on Leaving Bed

Lemon water	– without sugar, 1 glass
Or, a fruit	– anyone

Morning Breakfast

Coffee or tea	– without sugar, skimmed milk
Or, fruit juice	– 1 glass

Lunch

Vegetable soup	– ½ bowl
Chapattis	– thin ones without ghee 3
Dal	– 1 bowl
Or, fish or meat steamed	– about 100 gm
Salad	– as much as possible
Or, curd	– 1 bowl

Evening Breakfast

Lemon water	– without sugar
Or, tea	– skimmed milk, without sugar
Or, fruit juice	– 1 glass

Dinner

Chapattis	–	thin ones without ghee 4
Vegetable anyone	–	about 1 bowl
Or, rice boiled	–	about 100 gm
Salad (onion, tomato, carrot)	–	as much as possible
Green leafy vegetable	–	about 60 gm

□

88

Keep Cholesterol Under Control

Cholesterol is a form of fat. It falls under the category of derived fats. It is an element looking like wax and fat and is slippery. It is very essential for the body. The body produces cholesterol to meet its requirement by itself. There is no need for us to consume cholesterol in our diet. Cholesterol is found in our blood. It helps in generation of cell walls, sex hormones – estrogen and progesterone. It also functions as a messenger or transmitter in the nervous system of the body.

Cholesterol is found in all fatty foods. When such foods are consumed more than necessary, there is abundance of cholesterol in the body, which can be very harmful for the body.

To produce lipoprotein in the body, cholesterol merges with protein. This lipoprotein is of two types: the first is low density lipoprotein and the other is high density lipoprotein. In abbreviation or short form, they are also called LDL or HDL respectively.

As compared with HDL, LDL contains more fat. Due to this, this lipoprotein is light and can float in water. Due to this lipoprotein, cholesterol gets collected on the walls of blood vessels and veins. Due to excess of LDL in the blood, the blood vessels and capillaries become narrow, leading to obstruct the flow of blood. Generally, all heart ailments are related to this condition.

On the contrary, more quantity of HDL is good for health. HDL removes cholesterol from blood vessels and capillaries and delivers it into the liver, from where it is excreted.

To maintain the level of cholesterol in the body, it is essential that less fat-rich foods are consumed. The vegetable oils, such as obtained from soya bean, sunflower etc., have a lower amount of cholesterol. Therefore, you should avoid meat and milk, and should use vegetable oils obtained from vegetation.

□

89

Relation Between Fat and Obesity

Fat or lipid is an inseparable part of food and it is a good source of energy as well. As compared with other nutrients obtained from food, the fat collected in the body gives more calorie energy. Fat keeps body temperature or heat under control and also preserves soluble vitamins like A, D, K and E. Fat is also helpful in generation of hormones and clotting.

Fat is of two types – saturated and unsaturated.

Saturated fat remains solid even at normal temperature. It is found in animal products such as meat, butter, milk and some oils like coconut, palm, etc. This saturated fat becomes a factor in heart conditions and cancer.

Unsaturated fat is obtained from vegetable sources. This fat is in liquid form at room temperature. Unsaturated fat is of two types – poly-unsaturated and mono-unsaturated.

Poly-unsaturated fat contains sunflower, soya bean, cotton, til (gingelly), corn oils, etc., and mono-unsaturated fat contains peanut, olive, canola oils.

Normally, fat provides our body with heat and energy. When it is abundant in our food, the body accumulates extra fat in the body. This accumulated fat remains stored as an alternative for consumption during emergency.

When needed, the accumulated fat changes into carbohydrates and provides the body with energy.

In the body, fat is stored in fat cells. In the body of an ordinary person, there are about 300 trillion fat cells. The size of fat cells keeps changing. When there is more fat in the body, the number of fat cells increases further. If a person continues to consume more and more fat-rich foods, the fat accumulated in the body is not consumed or burnt, while the size and number of fat cells keep increasing. As a result, he gets obese in small duration of time.

□

90

Calorie Calculation of Different Foods

Per 100 gm

Food Items	*Calories*	*Food Items*	*Calories*
1. Grains			
Bajra	356	Corn (dry)	342
Rice	345	Wheat	341
Maida	348		
2. Dals (Pulses)			
Dal peeled	350	Gram, bean	346
Rajma (kidney bean)	340	Gram dal	360
3. Root Vegetables			
Carrot	47	Potato	97
Onion	59	Radish	17
4. Leafy Vegetables			
Chaulai (amaranth)	46	Methi (fenugreek), bathua	50
Spinach (palak)	26	Cabbage	27
Dhania (coriander)	44	Pudina	48
5. Non-vegetarian Foods			
Fish	111	Meat	173
Egg	194		

6. Milk Products

Curd	60	Buffalo milk	118
Buttermilk	15	Ghee	900
Paneer	292	Khoya	421

7. Fruits

Cheeku	118	Banana	79
Mango	70	Papaya	70
Apple	55	Guava	51
Orange	40		

□

91
Calorie and Obesity

The total calorie requirement for a person depends on different factors such as her age, sex and type of work he does. According to different surveys, the average daily calorie requirement for an ordinary man is about 2,500 calories, and that for an ordinary woman is about 2,100 calories. The more active a person is, the more calories she will need.

The elderly and old people spend less energy as compared to the youth. Therefore, the requirement of calorie goes down for them gradually. In the same way, a pregnant or lactating woman requires more calories than ordinary women, so they need to take a diet with more calories.

The chief factor of obesity depends on calorie intake. Suppose, a person requires 2,500 calorie energy a day. If he consumes food containing 2,500 calorie energy, his body will remain healthy, while maintaining a stable weight. Thus, such a person is able to consume all the calories he obtained from food. On the contrary, if a person consumes 500 calories more than his requirement, he will be able to get about 3,500 calories more in a week. Its simple outcome will be his increased weight. A person who consumes higher calorie diet will certainly become a victim of obesity.

If a person consumes more calorie diet but at the same time keeps working hard or takes exercise, his calorie energy will be burnt regularly. It will help him maintain a strong and shapely body.

About 50 calorie energy can be spent in a little time with simple measures. These can be enumerated as follows.

- Walk briskly or jog for 7 minutes.
- Dance for 8 minutes at a swift rate.
- Cycle for 15 minutes at a normal speed.
- Exercise lightly for 10 minutes.
- Skip rope for 6 minutes.
- Swim for 9 minutes.
- Play tennis for 12 minutes.

□

92

How to Prevent Increasing Fat

Obesity is directly related to fat. Fat cells present in the body keep increasing in size and number. With their continuous increase, the body inflates. Besides, the level of cholesterol also increases. As a consequence, ailments other than obesity also crop up. To get rid of all these ailments and problems, it is necessary to bring the amount of fat under control. If timely effort is not made in this direction, it can become quite a difficult task.

An ordinary person consumes about 45 kg of fat in an year. It is necessary for a healthy person to obtain, 30 percent of the required calorie from fat in the diet. Of this 30 percent fat in the diet, the part of saturated fat (that obtained from animals, coconut, palm etc.) should not be more than 10 percent. The remaining part should come from unsaturated fat (from soya bean, sunflower, etc.).

An obese person should not include any fatty food items in his diet. A varied diet prevents a person from getting obese. A varied diet means a diet which chiefly includes vegetables, fruits, grains, etc. It prevents him from getting obese. It also helps him obtain all the necessary nutrients.

In order to diminish the amount of fat in diet, the following recommendations can be kept in view:

- Minimise the use of food items made from ghee or oil. Use vegetable oil, but restrict its quantity to the minimum.
- The better thing to do is to boil, steam or roast than fry.
- Use milk without cream.

□

93

Use Fibre Diet

Fibre are like cleaning agents in our digestive system. They do not harm the body. When we eat fibrous foods and drink water, these fibres expand, but still remain soft. Passing along the walls of the food canal, they clean them. Doing this helps to remove toxins and unnecessary particles from the body for long. Fibrous foods stimulate the process of giving up food and clean the body.

According to health experts, constipation results from lack of fibre foods in diet. In constipation, the food gets stuck with the intestinal walls, which turns into toxins and these toxins can be the cause behind development of cancer in the intestines. Moreover, food items not containing fibre, such as meat, milk products etc. increase the level of fat and cholesterol in the body. It results into narrowing down of arteries, ultimately leading to heart problems. Refined carbohydrates have little quantity of fibrous food. They too play a vital role in developing obesity, diabetes, colon cancer and many other diseases.

Fibrous foods don't allow fat and cholesterol to get deposited in the body. This is very beneficial for people suffering from obesity, diabetes, heart disease, stone and repetitive constipation etc.

A normal person requires at least 30 gm of fibre diet daily. It is not necessary to add fibre in the diet. A balanced diet provides different types fibrous foods and required nutrition. A daily intake of fibre in the body has favourable impact on the health. The obese people should make it a specific point to include green vegetables, as palak (spinach), methi (fenugreek), bathua and beans, etc. The wheat flour should not be sieved. When the flour is not ground finely, it contains a sufficient quantity of bran. If you sieve this bran away, don't throw it, simply consume it with curd or mix it in the *halwa*.

If you love to have sweets, replace sweets and other sweet items with apple, pear, grapes, banana, alubukhara (plum) etc. All these fruits are good sources of fibre.

□

94

Dietary Myths

Honey is Best Medicine to do away Obesity

False. It is necessary to know that we don't get any nutrition from honey other than carbohydrates. Honey does not play any role in slimming down, whether it is taken mixed in simple water or in lemon water.

Drinking Water Early Morning is Beneficial in Slimming Down

False. Many people think that a glass of warm water in the morning immediately after waking up helps to reduce obesity. This myth is completely baseless. Some people opine that you can lose weight by about drinking 2 and a half litre of water during the whole day. This is also not the right fact. It can happen only when a person gives up all types of foods and subsists only on two and a half litre of water.

Cold Water Increases Obesity

False. Water is no food, so it cannot cause obesity. This fact is relevant to only fresh or refrigerated water. But beverages containing sweet or gas (aerated drinks) can generate obesity, such as syrups, sherbets, fruit juices etc.

Potato Stimulates Obesity

False. When compared with other food items, potato is responsible for less of obesity. In fact, a chapatti causes more weight gain than a piece of potato. Therefore, the myth that potatoes can increase obesity is meaningless.

Lemon Water is Helpful in Losing Weight

False. Many people believe that lemon water can help you lose weight, but they are not aware of the reality in depth. The truth remains that lemon water contains vitamin C, which helps to repair cells. This does not reduce any fat.

□

95

Get Rid of Dietary Myths

The olden beliefs in connection with the diet are not proper to follow in the modern context. These beliefs even tell that walking can also be harmful for the body.

How to drink water: Bottled and packaged water is quite prevalent these days, especially in cities. Bottled water is being sold as being more nutrient than ordinary tap water. But the truth remains that ordinary tap water contains more minerals

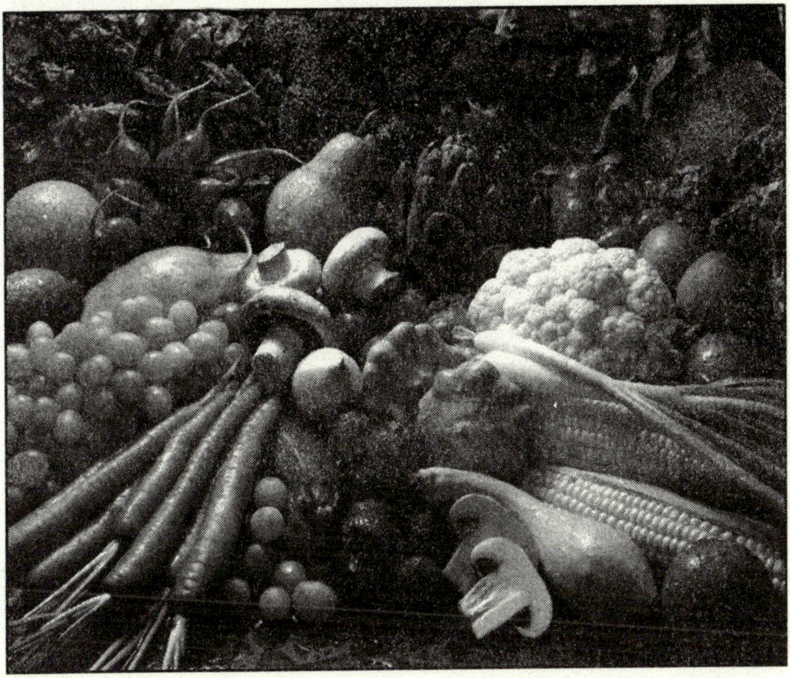

than bottled water. The most important fact to note is that bottled water contains more sodium which can result into high blood pressure.

How much fat is bad: In the present times, fat is being propagated as a foe to the health of man. This is true to a great extent. So a large number of people are influenced by this propaganda and keep away from all types of fatty foods. However, such a situation has a negative impact on their health. Our body requires at least 25 gm of fat and vitamins A, D, E, K and beta keratin which dissolve in fat. Therefore, it is essential that fat is consumed in a limited quantity.

How much of raw vegetables is good: You can hear every other person advising to eat raw vegetables as much as possible. Just think for a while, what will happen to a person who is incapable of digesting raw vegetables? Raw vegetables can do more harm than good to old people, children and those suffering from abdominal diseases. Therefore, it would be advisable to consume cooked vegetables.

How much of protein is good: It has been often seen that people compete so far as it pertains to consuming protein-rich diet; this is all more true in the case of players. The truth remains that players don't need extra protein, rather they require extra energy. Extra protein can be the cause of destruction of calcium present in the bones.

How much of salt is good: In our country, an ordinary person consumes as much as 17 gm of salt per day, which is as much as three times more than the prescribed limit of 5 gm. Therefore, the quantity of salt in diet should not exceed 5 gm. The people suffering from high blood pressure and heart diseases are advised to take 3 gm of salt a day.

□

96

Burn Calories to Stay Fit

Whatever activity you are engaged in, your body is continuously burning calories all the time, even when you are sleeping, when this rate is 50 to 85 calories an hour. This is the reason that it is essential to consume calories in a balanced manner in order to keep your body weight under control. This is natural that you burn more calories when you are doing some physical activity like walking. It simply means that you burn more calories while walking than you burn while sleeping, eating or sitting.

Keep in mind that as soon as you start to walk on foot, the capability of your body to do aerobics increases. With the help of your lungs, you start to breathe in more oxygen, which reaches your arteries and this helps in making your blood circulation proper. In this way, your blood reaches your muscles and cells in a proper quantity. Your body uses oxygen in order to manufacture energy. Oxygen plays a vital role in burning fat and this makes your body lose weight.

You might find it amazing but this remains true that walking on foot is the most reliable and safe way of losing weight. Crash diet and fad diet can make you feel that you are losing weight but such type of diet plan can in fact prove harmful and the weight lost in the initial stages can return with a vengeance. This fact has been proven beyond suspicion that those who try to lose weight by doing excessively hard work are tired after some time and they give up this practice and it results only in regaining their lost weight once again.

Walking to lose weight is considered to be the most reliable method. This method prevents the regaining of weight again. It is a slow process so the body gets habituated to this slow process. Those who walk regularly do not show any unprecedented or unusual increase in their body weight.

□

97

How to Choose Shoes for Walking

- Always buy good quality shoes for walking. Ensure that they fit well in the feet. Don't buy shoes on the basis of size only. Wear them to ensure that they fit well and pose no problem. If you are confident, buy them, else choose other. Remember that different brands and companies have varying sizes and the size can vary according to the pattern and style too.
- As you grow, the size of your feet also changes. If you measure your feet before buying shoes every time, it would help you greatly. Most people have one foot larger than the other one. While buying shoes, measure both feet. And then choose a pair which fits the larger foot.

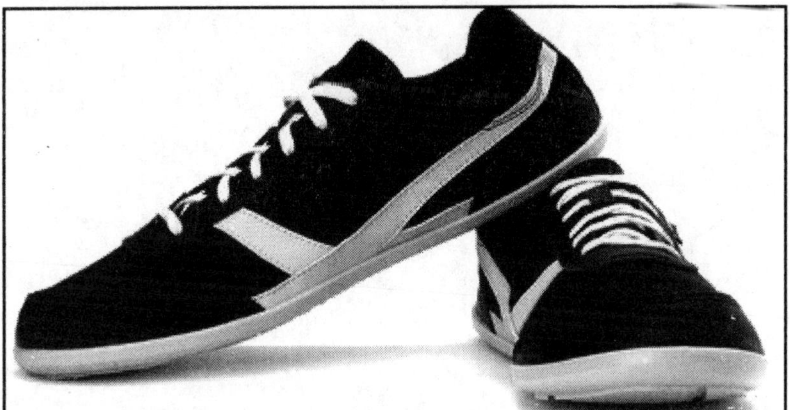

- Buy such shoes which are comfortable to your feet in relation to the size.
- If possible, buy shoes towards the evening; your feet are in their actual shape and size at that time.
- While buying, wear and stand up to see that they fit well. Ensure that your toe and the shoe wall have much space between them. There should be a little space there, else it would make walking a tough task. Also, the sole should be wide and comfortable so that you may not feel unnecessary pressure.
- Ensure that there is enough space in the shoes for the lower portion of your feet.
- Shoes must be made from such material which is comfortable to wear.
- Never buy tight shoes thinking they will expand later.
- Examine strength and structure of the sole and heel.
- Before you buy shoes, walk a few steps to ensure that you will not face any problem while using them.

□

98

Liposuction to Lose Weight Quickly

In the fast-paced busy life of modern times, people are starved for free time. Over and above, irregular daily routine and eating habits are also causing obesity to become a grave problem. However, you can lose weight by the liposuction technique.

We are left with little time due to our busy schedule in office and home and we are unable to look after ourselves. We tend to eat what we may lay hands on. We don't even stop to think what effect it will have on our body. In fact, such type of food becomes the chief factor of our obesity.

What Liposuction Is

This is a technique of cosmetic surgery, called lipectomy With this, the additional fat is sucked out of different parts of the body in order to make it shapely and attractive. Under this process, in the hidden places of our body, small holes are made in order to suck out additional fat with the help of special equipment. The time needed for this process depends on the quantity of fat in the body.

Where to Use It

The liposuction technique is chiefly used on abdomen, hips, thighs, arms, face and thorax. Both men and women undergo this process to bring their bodies in shape. This surgery is used to suck out fat from different body parts.

Approaching Liposuction

If you are thinking of undergoing the process of liposuction, you should go to a qualified plastic surgeon. This is a type of surgery, so this operation should be performed by an experienced and qualified surgeon. At first, consult a surgeon if this process is good for your body or not. Also find out if this process will prove successful on you; also find out the problems that you are likely to face before and after the process. If you are aware of all these facts, you will not be worried while undertaking this process.

After Surgery

After the surgery, there may be some excretion from holes, but there is nothing to worry about. Sometimes you may have complaints of swelling and pain, which will get right with time. Continue to undergo medical checkup after the surgery too. This surgery will help you get a good figure but you have to undertake physical exercise and have control over your diet in order to maintain that attractive figure.

□

99

Ayurveda to Lose Weight

According to ayurveda, being under- or over-weight is the symptom of imbalance between Vata, Pitta and Kafa. If your diet is not balanced in metabolic terms, the problem of weight is sure to arise.

Kafa is blamed for obesity. Of course, you can find other defects/imbalances in an obese person too.

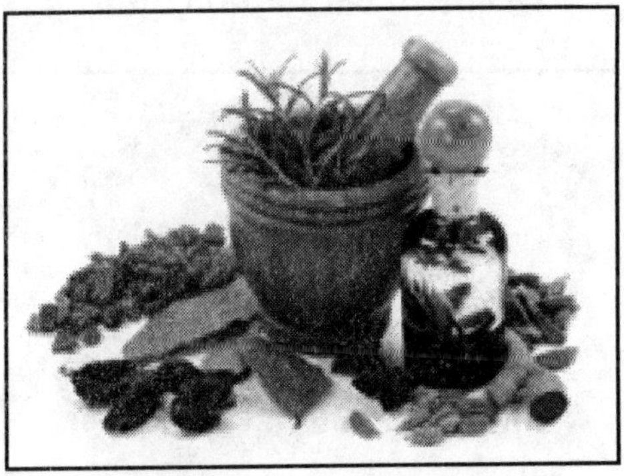

Under ayurveda, strategy to lose weight is formulated after due evaluation of the body and mind of the individual. The procedure for treatment is defined on the basis of imbalance.

Ayurvedic Advice

- Avoid things as may be convenient to you and follow a balanced lifestyle.
- Include those food items in diet which help in digestion such as ginger, papaya, mango, pineapple, etc.
- Have ginger tea two-three times a day for improvement in digestion. Also observe fasting once a week.
- Include jeera, mustard, red chilli and black pepper in diet.
- Exercise regularly.

□

100

Control Eating Useless Things

Many researchers opine that there can be physiological as well as emotional causes behind eating improper food items. When a person is being stimulated to eat ice-cream, pizza or other junk food, it is not at all necessary for him to be stimulated by appetite only.

Desire to Eat Carbohydrates: Low blood sugar can cause

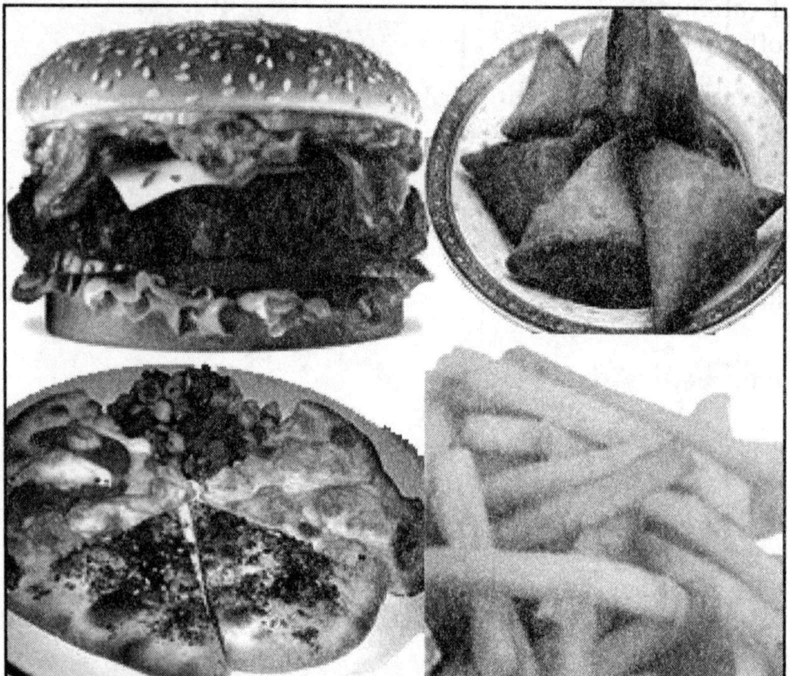

a desire to eat sweet, cake, chips, cracker and the like. Such a situation arises when you stay hungry for a long time or are emotionally depressed. Women can face this situation before the onset of menstruation cycle. To prevent the evil effect of carbohydrates, fruits, vegetables and grains can be consumed as an alternative. A person can also be helped by consuming protein-rich foods or toned milk.

Desire to Eat Salt: A continuous situation of stress can lead to a desire to eat pickle, chips and other salted products. Lemon water and herbal tea can be opted for as an alternative. Including fresh fruits help to reduce the desire to eat salted things.

Desire to Consume Caffeine: Caffeine is found in products like tea, coffee and cold drinks. Some people are mentally as well as physically habituated of having caffeine and when they don't consume it, they feel headache, fatigue, unconsciousness and peevishness etc., and this makes them consume more sugar. To do away with this habit, the quantity of caffeine should be decreased gradually and caffeine-free coffee, herbal tea, etc. should be consumed.

□

101

Importance of Protein in Weight Loss

Protein is helpful in maintaining a proper balance of water in the body. Some people are in fact not obese but they have extra amount of water in their bodies. The body tissues have the capability to hold on to water. If you push your finger through the obese part of such a person, a pit or depression will be formed, which will still be there for a moment after you have removed your finger. Such obesity is generally due to lack of protein in the body. When water gets collected in the body, the situation is called 'oedema'. If the deficiency of protein is fulfilled with a balanced diet, such looseness in the body disappears after some time.

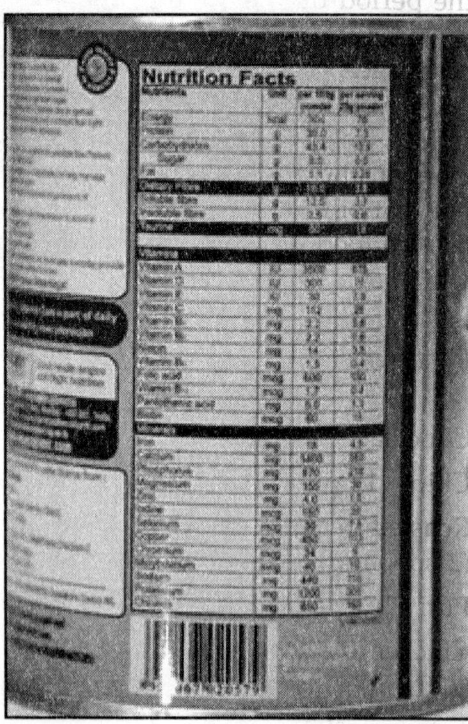

All types of proteins are formed by the compound of about 24 different types of chemical units. All these chemical units contain nitrogen in a specific quantity. These chemical units are known as amino acids. As different letters are arranged in different ways to form millions of words; much in the same manner, amino acids too join together in different ways to form different types of proteins.

The proteins consumed by us in diet are broken into amino acids. These amino acids link together like bricks to form necessary protein for the living being. All 24 types of amino acids cannot be found in our diet at any one time. Only 8 of these amino acids are such which the body needs regularly. The rest of them can be formed by the body by itself. No hormone, enzyme or protein can be formed in the body without amino acids (extremely essential for different physiological processes).

It is not enough to have a diet equipped with protein. It is also necessary to consume protein of good quality.

Generally, the people aspiring to lose weight need much protein. If the body is not supplied with required protein during the period of diet control, the body tissues are deprived of proper nutrition. Lack of proteins only causes weakness and it cannot lead to weight loss.

If you keep taking protein in your balanced diet in order to lose weight, no harm will be caused to your body. In this manner, the realized weight loss will be that of only fat and not that of health. If you shift to protein-rich food in place of fat-rich food, you certainly will be able to lose weight.

Chips vs. Papad

Food Items	*Kilo Calorie*	*Alternative Food*	*Kilo Calorie*
Chocolate cookies	175	Cream cracker	76
Chips (12 pieces)	210	Papad	165
Roasted peanut (2 spoonful)	170	Roasted gram	70
Puri (2)	200	Chapatti (2 dry)	100
Chicken biryani (100 gm cooked)	275	White rice	100

Cooked veg (paneer)	200		
Dal makhani (1 spoon cream)	210		
Cream soup (1 spoon ghee, 1 spoon cream)	115		
Cola (1 bottle)	180		75
Russian salad	184		
Chicken fry (1 leg piece)	370	Chicken tandoori	75

Eat and Run

Glance through this table. Next time your child demands any of these things, tell him which exercise or activity he will have to do and for how much time. Before he think to eat any of these things, he will think thrice, so says Pratigya Bali.

Food Items	*Quantity*	*Kilo Calorie*	*Activity/Exercise Required to Spend Calorie*
Pav-bhaji	1 plate	600	40 minute running (8-10 km)
Bhelpuri	1 plate	370	30 minute swimming
Cheese pizza	100 gm	225	30 minute badminton
French fry	15 pieces	165	20 minute cycling (15 km)
Cashew nut	12 pieces	149	20 minute cycling (15 km)
Gulab jamun	2 pieces	250	20 minute aerobics (continuously)
Chocolate ice-cream	1 small cup	290	1 hour table tennis
Chocolate cake	1 piece	200	20 minute football

Don't Let Children Gain Weight

- Teach your children to eat food slowly.
- If thirsty, don't give them Coke, give water instead.
- Decrease on snacks.
- Teach them games and sports (tennis, badminton etc.)
- Reward the child to bring about positive change in health in order to form positive habits.
- Encourage the child to take part in games at school.

Behavioural Reform in Obesity: Initial Objective

- Start with light adjustments.
- Make specific goals, for example:
  - Reduce chips to half.
  - While going to market, don't add to the list.
  - Stop buying chocolate from the neighbourhood shop.
- If you fulfil your goal, reward yourself, but not in the form of edible things.

The Beauty of Our Dreams Determines Our Future

- Let everybody be happy.
- Let everybody be healthy.
- Let us pray for the well-being of everybody.
- Let no person suffer.

Self-help

- None knows you better than you.
- None can eat for you.
- None can lose weight for you.
- None can think for you.
- None can stop you from forming bad habits.
- None can form good habits in you.
- None can eat medicine for you.
- Only YOU can change yourself, none else can change you.

Behavioural Diagnosis

Methods to Stimulation Control

- Eat thrice a day.
- Fix the times and place of eating.
- Place food on the table and sit down to eat.
- Stop the habit of not keeping an eye on what you are eating.
- Take a smaller plate for food.
- Place the food on table and eat slowly.
- Stop a while after having tasted a food item.
- Avoid the food items that create problems for you.
- Avoid frying with more calories.
- Serve food in small quantities.
- Avoid eating the food served the second time.

Behavioural Diagnosis

Methods of Strengthening

- Reward yourself on change of behaviour and not change in weight.
- Don't take food items as reward.
- Choose conspicuous items, such as money or clothing.
- Reward immediately after a goal has been achieved.

Dieticians advise to consume the food as follows.

Nutrition Pyramid

Food Items	*Nutrition Pyramid*	*Nutrients Obtained*
Fat sugar	Eat with restriction	Energy
Milk products	Have normal quantity (2-3 times)	Protein
Fish, Meat,	Eat normally	
Pulses, Eggs	(2-3 times)	Calcium, iron, magnesium, vitamin B, tissue-forming minerals; these strengthen the skeleton.

Vegetables (2-3 times)	Eat much	
Fruits (2-4 times)	(5-9 times)	Minerals; maintain skin, hair, nails, blood and soft tissues. Vitamins are good for ligaments, blood, bones, tissues, eyes, brain.
Chapatti/Bread, Grains/Rice	Eat sufficiently (6–11 times)	Carbohydrates provide energy for proper motion of body and organs; give energy for physical activities.

Pyramid of Physical Activity

Avoid watching television, internet surfing, talking on phone, sitting more than 30 minutes, playing computer games.

Sedentary Activities

Yoga, exercise, spreading hands and feet, lifting light weight, push-ups, bench press.

Lifting light weight thrice a week, turning abdomen, cough rage, etc.

Power Exercise and Physical Flexibility

Walking, cycling, skating, climbing stairs, swimming.

Playing tennis, dancing, long-distance walking etc. – 5 days a week.

Aerobics and Recreational Exercises

Whenever possible, walk. Walk briskly while going to take bus (5-6 km an hour). If possible, get down the bus one stop short of your destination while going to office, school or market. Stroll in the colony at lunch time. Clean your room. Change to stairs in place of the lift. Keep exercising while watching television.

Behavioural Improvement for Obesity: Goal Setting

Long-term Objectives

- Don't buy the things you should not eat.
- Include prohibited food items in your diet in a very controlled manner (for example, chocolate only after lunch on Sunday afternoon).
- Eat thrice a day, in addition to two snacks daily.
- Eat something between two meals.
- Avoid eating after meals.

□□□